6 WEEKS
To A
TOXIC -FREE
BODY

6 WEEKS
To A
TOXIC -FREE
BODY

A Step By Step Program On
How To Achieve A Toxic-Free Body

By
Dean D. Kimmel

Foreword by Norman Wolk, M.D.

CORBIN HOUSE
New York

Although the author and publisher have extensively researched all sources to ensure the accuracy and completeness of the information provided, we cannot assume responsibility for errors, inaccuracies, omissions or any other inconsistency herein. The information provided in this book is intended to educate you, the reader, about good health habits. It is not a substitute for personalized medical care. Please consult your physician before following the recommendations made herein.

Library of Congress Cataloging-in-Publication Data

Kimmel, Dean D.
   6 weeks to a toxic-free body / Dean D. Kimmel. — 1st ed.
   p. cm.
   Includes bibliographical references and index.
   ISBN 0-9621446-2-2 (pbk.)
   1. Food—Toxicology—Health aspects. 2. Food additives—Health aspects. 3. Food contamination—Health aspects. 4. Nutrition.
I. Title. II. Title: Six weeks to a toxic-free body.
RA1258.K56 1992
615.9'54—dc20   90-80854

Published by
Corbin House
227 Corbin Place
Brooklyn, New York 11235
Printed in the United States of America.

THE FIRST WEALTH IS HEALTH.

-Ralph Waldo Emerson

CONTENTS

ACKNOWLEDGMENTS

I wish to express my heartfelt gratitude to Norman Wolk, M.D., for carefully reviewing this book and for giving me invaluable advice, and lots of encouragement and support. I am also very grateful for the time he gave me from his very demanding schedule.

My sincere gratitude and thanks to Herbert M. Garcia, M.D., Joel Fuhrman, M.D., Avraham Y. Henoch, M.D., and Anthony J. Penepent, M.D., for carefully reviewing this book and for giving helpful comments.

Special thanks to Joseph Reed for sharing with me his keen insights on Natural Hygiene. His vast knowledge of Natural Hygiene and healthful living never ceases to amaze me.

Many thanks to Bernice and Shirley Davison, Directors of the Health Oasis; Douglas N. Graham, D.C., Director of Club Hygiene; Keki R. Sidwa, D.O., President of the British Natural Hygiene Society and Director of the Shalimar Retreat; Susan Taylor and the American Natural Hygiene Society; Jo Willard, President of Natural Hygiene Inc.; Rhoda Mozorosky, Director of the Umpqua House; and Philip Martin, D.C., for providing me with recipes. I thank Carlson Wade, literary agent and author of *Eat Away Illness* and *Nutritional Therapy*; Roger Field, former health and science editor at the NBC radio network; and Stanley S. Bass, D.C., for their advice.

FOREWORD

Radiant health, boundless energy, abiding strength, enduring vitality, profound well being; these are the qualities all who seek "the good life" earnestly desire. Beyond the popular goals of financial security, material comforts and the achievement of personal potential, we realize that none are truly possible without freedom from disease.

As the final years of the twentieth century draw to a close, humanity finds itself at the threshold of an uncertain future. For many of us, the threat of war, disease, social disintegration and environmental pollution have robbed our sense of hope and confidence in tomorrow. Not too long ago, fresh air, clean water, good untainted food, were all easily obtainable. Yet today, in a world relentlessly pursuing the illusions of progress, these simple but essential products have become as rare as the perfect jewel.

Dean Kimmel, in his exciting breakthrough book, *6 Weeks To A Toxic-Free Body*, invites us to reflect upon our modern times and the triple threats of cancer, heart disease, and stroke. We are introduced to the reality of a poisoned world, and the very real possibility that we can affect our future for the good. Armed with the wisdom of the ages, we are beckoned to discover that a good, healthy, and happy life free from debilitating and devastating disease can be ours.

From the beginning of time, humanity has sought a place where lasting well being and confident hope in the future is an ever present reality. I urge you to spend 6 Weeks on a journey that can change your life and restore your faith in a brighter tomorrow. Join Dean Kimmel and his many readers on this extraordinary adventure, and recover precious assurance that the best is yet to come.

Norman Wolk, M.D.

INTRODUCTION

The term toxic literally means poisonous. Toxemia is the condition that results from long term exposure to toxic, or poisonous substances. Most of us, needlessly, are exposed to toxic substances on a daily basis. From the air we breathe, from the job we work, to the food we eat, we are living in a country that is laden with toxic substances.

It seems as though there is no escape from toxic substances. Toxic chemicals surround us. What can we do? How can we lower our exposure to toxins? And what can we do if our bodies already exceed safe limits? Is there a safe, effective method for eliminating toxins from the body?

6 Weeks To A Toxic-Free Body shows how you can achieve a toxic-free body in 6 weeks or less, by making smart, sensible changes in your lifestyle. The guidelines presented are for everybody. No matter what age you are, you can benefit. No matter what physical condition you are in, you can benefit.

This book also discusses why the foods we eat are leading causes of toxemia. Heart disease and cancer are, in many instances, directly caused by the foods we eat. By emphasizing a dietary approach, *6 Weeks To A Toxic-Free Body* shows how these and other diseases and illnesses can be prevented.

Here's to a healthful, toxic-free body!

1

FIGHTING PESTICIDES, INSECTICIDES, AND OTHER TOXIC CHEMICALS IN OUR FOOD SUPPLY

It is only recently that large numbers of American consumers became fed up with chemical pesticides, insecticides, fungicides, and herbicides. Hazardous chemical pesticides have been in commercial use by food growers before World War II, and the health dangers have long been much overlooked and ignored by the public. Thanks to the tremendous clout of the media, which in recent years has become more concerned with the environment, and thanks to the growing number of influential consumer advocate groups, the dangers of chemical pesticides became an issue that could no longer be overlooked or ignored.

Consumer advocate groups, in their fight against the widespread use of harmful pesticides, have made an enormous impact on the public. Consumer advocate groups, especially the following: Americans for Safe Food, Natural Resources Defense Council, Mothers and Others for Pesticide Limits, and the National Academy of Sciences, have been largely credited with educating Americans about the health dangers of chemical pesticides. The Alar incident in 1989 is an example of what type of impact these consumer advocate groups can have. In their campaign against Alar, a chemical applied on apples to increase ripening and help preserve crispness, Alar became a household word.

According to a report published by the National Resources Defense Council (NRDC), Alar (also known as daminozide) is a carcinogen (cancer-causing substance) which is especially hazardous to children.[1] Alar residues were found on all varieties of apples except Granny Smith.

Alar and all pesticides pose a greater health threat to children than adults because the immune system in children is not yet fully developed. Also, children take in more fruits and vegetables to fulfill the enormous energy demands of their growing bodies. The NRDC estimates that at least 17 percent or 3 million preschoolers (ages 1-5) are exposed to neurotoxic organophosphate insecticides from just eating raw fruits and vegetables.[2] According to the NRDC, the average child consumes six times as much fruit as the average adult.[3] The average toddler consumes 18 times as much apple juice and 31 times as much apple sauce as the average adult.[4] The NRDC claims that children receive up to 400 percent more exposure to pesticides than adults do.[5] In 1989, as a direct result of these findings, schools across America banned apples from being served in cafeterias.

Despite drastic measures taken by apple growers such as placing full-page advertisements in major newspapers to convince the public that commercially grown apples are safe to eat, in 1989, sales of apples plummeted. Even a last ditch attempt to boost sales by offering incredibly low prices, failed to win over consumers. Americans, in 1989, by and large stayed away from apples. The link between Alar and apples in the minds of Americans spelled disaster for apple growers. Apple growers posted one of their worst years in sales on record. Due to public pressure, virtually all apple growers in the United States voluntarily agreed not to apply Alar on future apple crops. With the fear of Alar gone, apples made their return to school cafeterias.

Janet Hathaway of the NRDC said, "We definitely made the apple industry think."[6] She added, "The industry is now interested in reducing its pesticide use. They are starting to collect data on chemicals themselves."[7]

Other harmful chemicals that have been highly publicized in recent years include ethylene bisdithiocarbamates (EBDCs) such as aldicarb, maneb, and mancozeb. Aldicarb, a very deadly insecticide, used on potatoes and imported bananas, was viewed by the Environmental Protection Agency's (EPA) pesticide division as an unreasonable health risk. Toxicologists maintain that thousands of infants and children are exposed to high levels of residues of aldicarb in bananas and potatoes. According to the EPA, each day 26,000 to 81,500 children under the age of 6 are exposed to aldicarb in amounts which present a risk of getting ill from eating potatoes.[8] Tiny amounts of aldicarb residues in potatoes and bananas may cause stomach cramps, nausea, headaches, nervous disorders, blurred vision, and elevated heart rates.[9] Toxicologists claim that one drop of aldicarb absorbed through the skin can kill an adult.[10] Aldicarb is so deadly that farmers do not risk spraying it on crops. For safety measures, aldicarb is applied as a granule.

Aldicarb was developed in 1965 and became commercially available in the U.S. in 1970 by the Union Carbide Corporation. Union Carbide originally planned to promote aldicarb as a chemical that killed insects that fed on cotton and other inedible crops. Experiments with this chemical, however, proved to be equally effective in controlling pests on food crops. The insecticide is made from methyl isocyanate, the chemical responsible for killing over 2,000 people and injuring thousands more in the December 1984 leak at the Union Carbide plant in Bhopal, India.[11]

Since its first use on potato farms in 1974, in Suffolk County, New York, aldicarb has been met with disastrous results. The widespread use of aldicarb has contaminated many water supplies. In 1979, Suffolk County, New York was the site of a major contamination. In Suffolk County, aldicarb in underground water was found to be 50 times higher than the safety level established by the EPA.[12] In 1980, 19 wells in Wisconsin were found to be contaminated with aldicarb.[13] In 1983, aldicarb was found in wells in Florida, California, New Jersey, Massachusetts, and upstate New York.[14] In 1985, California was the site of a major aldicarb contamination. Millions of watermelons contaminated with aldicarb were destroyed in California after a thousand illnesses were reported.[15]

In 1989, after EPA investigations, aldicarb, also known by its trade name, Temik, has been detected in water supplies in 22 states.[16] Aldicarb has also been used extensively in the two largest potato-producing states, Idaho and Washington. Due to pressure from consumer organizations, especially the National Resources Defense Council, aldicarb is no longer used on potato crops in the United States. In 1990, the manufacturer of aldicarb, Rhone Poulenc Ag Company, announced that it will no longer sell aldicarb for use on potatoes.[17]

Since aldicarb has not been banned for use on bananas and coffee, be careful when purchasing bananas and coffee. Though not widely available, it is preferable to purchase bananas and coffee grown in the U.S. As you will see later in this chapter, imported foods often contain much higher residues of harmful pesticides than foods grown in this country. It should be pointed out that the best bananas and coffee, as is the case for all foods, are those which have been organically grown (more on that later).

Ethylene bisdithiocarbamates (better known as EBDCs) are chemicals used to kill fungus and bacteria. Some farmers claim if EBDCs are not applied to crops, fungus and bacteria can develop unsightly spots on leaves and stems, or ruin entire fields of fruit and vegetables. Out of the five EBDCs, two, maneb and mancozeb, are among the most widely used fungicides by Florida vegetable growers. According to the chief of the Special Review Branch of the EPA, Janet L. Auerbach, maneb and mancozeb are carcinogenic. Using a new method of detecting pesticide residues in vegetables, the EPA found the risk of developing cancer from the EBDCs is 2 cases in 100,000 people.[18] This risk factor is a rate 20 times higher than the established federal limit.[19] Such findings prompted the EPA to consider setting more stringent guidelines governing the use of EBDCs.

Because of carcinogens associated with EBDCs, increased negative public perception of chemical pesticides, and the development of chemical-free pesticides being tested in California, Arizona, and other desert states, Florida farmers are becoming aware of the fact that chemical pesticide use is a threat to their livelihood-physically and economically. To keep up with the times, Florida growers are experimenting with a number of new methods to reduce the need for chemicals. New methods include surveying fields for insects and diseases, planting hardier varieties of crops, and using natural pesticides that use bacteria to kill insect larvae.

Alar, aldicarb, maneb, and mancozeb represent only a tiny fraction of the harmful chemicals used in our food supply. In 1988, the EPA classified more than 70 of approximately 360 pesticides licensed for use on food, as suspected human carcinogens.[20] What about pesticides which are in use today that were introduced before licensing laws were enacted? What harm do they cause? There are hundreds of chemicals used in our food supply that have never been tested for health effects. For example, nerve poisons are being used as pesticides even though they have never been tested for neurological effects.[21] A study performed by the National Academy of Sciences revealed that 64 percent of pesticides now in use have not even been minimally tested for their toxic effects.[22] Furthermore, tests commonly used by the Food and Drug Administration can only detect residues of 107 of the approximate 360 pesticides.[23]

Here is an added blow to the consumer: Pesticides banned from use in this country are sold by the American government to foreign countries, only to return to us in the food we import. Ethically, the U.S. finds nothing wrong with this practice. And the governments of many foreign countries, especially those in underdeveloped countries, have little or no laws regulating the use of chemical pesticides.

Third world countries are paying dearly for "modernizing" their agriculture. The United Nations Food and Agricultural Organization found that very toxic pesticides are widely available in at least 85 developing countries.[24] The United

Nations revealed that 80 of these countries have no adequate agency that approves, registers, or monitors pesticides.[25] Most third world countries are also not informed on the the hazards of pesticide use, and they do not have people trained to evaluate them.

The World Health Organization estimated that about a million people suffer acute poisoning from pesticides every year and many of them are farmers in the third world.[26] The organization reported that pesticides cause about 20,000 deaths a year.[27] According to an article in *The New York Times*, "World pesticide sales have nearly doubled since the mid-1970's to nearly $18 billion a year, and much of this growth has taken place in the third world."[28]

The New York Times article also says, "The United States annually exports about 500 million pounds of pesticides that are banned, restricted or not licensed for domestic use."[29] Under American regulations, a manufacturer is required by law to notify the Environmental Protection Agency about shipments. The EPA is responsible for informing receiving countries about pesticides. However, Congressional hearings in May of 1989 revealed that only 10 percent of the exports are filed with the EPA. It was found that most exporters took advantage of an EPA loophole that exempts filing if the pesticides are similar to other approved pesticides.[30] Since the U.S. Food and Drug Administration only samples 1 to 2 percent of all imports arriving in this country, it is best to avoid imported food.[31]

Although fruits and vegetables have received much press coverage for containing harmful residues of chemical pesticides, meats, poultry, eggs, and dairy products are also heavily contaminated. It has been found that pesticides and other toxic substances accumulate in foods high in fat. Meats, poultry, eggs, and dairy products (foods which are notoriously high in fat) contain more pesticide residues and other contaminants than foods low in fat such as fruits and vegetables.

According to Dr. Edward L. Menning, director of the National Association of Federal Veterinarians, at least 60 percent of meats, poultry and fish sold at retail may be contaminated.[32] For example, more than half the chickens sold in the U.S. may contain salmonella.[33] And there is a 1-in-50 chance of encountering an egg contaminated with salmonella.[34]

Commercially sold meats, poultry, eggs, and dairy products contain high levels of pesticides and fungicides, as well as harmful injections of growth hormones, artificial coloring and flavoring agents, antibiotics, and other drugs.

Studies in the U.S. have shown that 100 percent of poultry, 90 percent of pigs and veal calves, and 60 percent of all cattle are routinely fed antibiotics.[35] However, less than one out of every million animals slaughtered in the U.S. is tested for toxic chemical residues.[36] The United States General Accounting Office has identified 143 drugs and pesticides that are likely to leave residues in raw meat and poultry.[37] Out of these 143 drugs and pesticides, 42 are known or suspected carcinogens, 20 of these may cause birth defects, and 6 may cause mutations.[38]

It is ironic that the United States Department of Agriculture (USDA) reassured Americans for years that meat was safe to eat by stamping it with "Choice," "Prime," or "U.S. No. 1 USDA." It was then proven that the ink, Violet Dye No. 1, was found to be carcinogenic.[39] Recently the U.S. government banned this dye from being stamped on meat.[40]

Dr. Michael Klaper, an expert on the health hazards of animal consumption, provides this grim account: "Animals get cancers, especially if they are fed hormones to make them fatter, if they graze on lands contaminated with sprayed crops, and they are fed grains that have been sprayed with pesticides and spoil retardants. The cows get the cancers. When a cow with a cancer is slaughtered, it comes down the assembly line, and that carcass, if it has a cancer, should be pulled off the line. The carcasses come by very quickly. The cancer tissue is ground up into hamburger, and it goes right on by, no-one will ever see it, it just gets made into sausage."[41]

Poultry is faced with similar problems that afflict beef. Chickens, like cows, get cancers from the contaminants fed to them. The most common form of cancer in chickens is lymphoma, cancer of the lymph glands. A virus (in chicken droppings and dust) spread lymphomas from one chicken to another.[42] According to Dr. Klaper, when the tissue from a person with lymphoma is put under a microscope it is identical to the lymphoma found in chickens. He claims the more meat, and especially chicken, eaten, the higher the rates of lymphoma.[43]

Although the health dangers of eating meat injected with growth hormones have been well documented, Americans, by and large have done nothing to protest this practice. Europeans, on the other hand, have taken measures against meat treated with growth hormones. Consumer groups, especially in Germany, have successfully educated Europeans about the dangers of meat injected with hormones such as testosterone, estradiol, and progesterone, and the synthetic hormones zeranol and trenbolone. In 1985, the 12-nation European Economic Community (EEC) prohibited hormone use within the EEC nations. Heeding to the demands of European farmers, the EEC, in 1989 banned imported meat treated with growth hormones. This action spelled bad news for American beef producers, since $100 million in U.S. exports would be lost annually.[44] As a result of the European ban on American meat, the U.S. has threatened to retaliate by imposing high tariffs on imported food from Europe. Falling prey to American agribusiness interests, the U.S. government is unwilling to ban hormone-treated meat.

Some people become aware of the dangers inherent to eating meat, and switch to fish. Fish is often recommended by health professionals for its beneficial fatty acids, such as Omega-3's, which are said to lower one's cholesterol level. When people switch from eating meat to eating fish, little do they know they are trading one set of problems for another; fish consumption can be just as harmful as meat consumption.

Chemical pesticides used to spray crops, seep into lakes, streams, rivers, and oceans inhabited by fish. Factories routinely discharge heavy metals such as cadmium and mercury into these bodies of water.[45] With each rainfall, agricultural chemicals and industrial pollutants contaminate lakes, streams, rivers, and oceans. Fish living in these waters absorb large amounts of contaminants and become highly toxic. Health expert Dr. Michael Klaper states: "I don't know any place where you could analyze fish flesh on this planet any longer and not find traces of hydrocarbons, of heavy metals, of pollutants of all sorts."[46]

Young, small fish contain fewer contaminants than old, large fish. And in general, fattier fishes contain more contaminants. The exception is salmon. Even though they have a high fat content, salmon are not highly contaminated (except those originating from very polluted waters such as the Great Lakes).[47]

Since toxic chemicals accumulate in the fatty tissue, skinning and proper trimming can help reduce the risks of eating contaminated fish. The skin, the belly flap, and the fatty (brown-colored) streaks at the top or center of the fillet should be trimmed. The green-colored tomalley in lobster or the "mustard" in blue crabs should not be eaten because these are sites where toxic chemicals are concentrated.[48] Also, it may be wise to discard the innards (entrails) and gills; it is extremely dangerous to eat internal organs of potentially contaminated fish.[49]

When people consume contaminated fish, toxins accumulate in various parts of the body. Toxins accumulate in fat tissue, muscle, and bone.[50] After a decade or so, consumption of contaminated fish can cause birth defects, cancer, neurological diseases, and other degenerative diseases.[51]

Laws governing the safety of the fish we eat are poorly regulated. There are no national standards for warnings about contaminated fish, and there are no nationwide rules for sampling and testing. Some states test whole fish; some test fish without the skin or entrails. Those states that test fish without the entrails are short-changing the public. It is important to test fish containing entrails because this is the part of the fish where toxins concentrate.[52]

As for the testing itself, there are no uniform guidelines for collecting and handling samples. And as a further indicator of lax control, the quality of laboratories that test fish can vary greatly.[53]

States that have the most fish consumption advisories (which warn against eating fish from certain waters) are not indications that these states have the most contaminated waters. It could mean such states have the best monitoring policies. Fourty-four states have fish consumption advisories. The six states that do not are Alaska, Idaho, Iowa, North Dakota, Oregon, and Wyoming.

Conditions surrounding eggs and dairy products are deplorable. Egg-laying hens are given artificially colored feed for the purpose of making the color of the pale yolks more attractive.[54] Some egg producers add chemicals such as arsenic to increase maturation and stimulate egg production.[55] Dairy products may contain residues of chemicals or drugs used in the feed. According to Debra Lynn Dadd, author of *The Nontoxic Home*, "All milk sold in the United States today contains pesticides; no milk is free from them because all grazing lands are still contaminated with banned pesticides such as DDT."[56]

Chemicals are indeed deadly. The EPA reports that chemical residues on food pose the third greatest cancer risk in America today.[57] The National Academy of Sciences estimates that there are 20,000 cancer deaths a year due to pesticides alone.[58]

Pesticides have been linked to cancers and birth defects among farmers, farmworkers, and their families. Millions of farmers who use chemicals are jeopardizing their lives. Medical studies have shown that Kansas farmers develop Non-Hodgkins Lymphoma at 6 times the rate of the general population.[59] Children in the large farming community of San Joaquin, California have a cancer rate 8 times the norm.[60]

The implications from chemical use are far reaching. From the air we breathe, to the foods we eat, to the oceans we swim in, chemicals know no boundaries. At an unprecedented rate, chemicals are causing widespread havoc to the environment. Our ground water, rivers, and lakes are streaming with pollution. According to the EPA, ground water contamination exists in 41 states.[61] The worst ground water contamination exists in the nation's croplands where

22.3 billion pounds of nitrogen fertilizer and 850 million pounds of agricultural chemicals are used each year.[62]

Such pollution is a disgrace considering the fact that there are a multitude of safe alternatives to agricultural chemicals. The National Academy of Sciences conducted a study and reported that farmers who apply little or no chemicals to crops can be as productive as those who use pesticides and synthetic fertilizers. The National Academy of Sciences has recommended that Congress and the Department of Agriculture change Federal subsidy programs that encourage overuse of agricultural chemicals. The Academy said that it was seeking to reverse Federal policies that, for more than 40 years have been focused on increasing the productivity of crop and livestock farms through heavy use of pesticides, drugs, and synthetic fertilizers.[63]

The Academy committee said, "Well-managed alternative farms use less synthetic chemical fertilizers, pesticides and antibiotics without necessarily decreasing, and, in some cases, increasing per-acre crop yields and the productivity of livestock systems."[64]

The report "Alternative Agriculture" issued by the National Academy of Sciences, also said, "Wider adoption of proven alternative systems would result in ever greater economic benefits to farmers and environmental gains for the nation."[65]

At present, food distributors are not required by law to inform consumers of foods containing pesticides. Farmers, and in many instances food distributors, know what chemicals are applied. For fear of losing sales, many farmers and food distributors are unwilling to share such information.

The health hazards associated with commercially sold foods, foods laden with dangerous levels of pesticides, insecticides, fungicides, herbicides, hormone stimulants, and antibiotics, help explain why organically grown food is so popular.

The term "organic" is generally defined as foods which have been grown using ecologically sound methods of farming. Chemical pesticides or synthetic fertilizers are not used. In many instances, organic fruits and vegetables look different from conventional (regular) produce. Sometimes organic produce may not be as aesthetically appealing as conventional produce. Do not hold this against organic produce.

Pesticides are often used for the chief purpose of preventing blemishes on fruits and vegetables. For example, a survey conducted among citrus growers found that 76 to 100 percent of their pesticides were mainly used to protect the appearance of the fruit.[66] It is truly disturbing that pesticides are being used for the sole purpose of maintaining a fruit's appearance. And it is a sad fact that consumers have been taught that the best fruits and vegetables are those which look picture-perfect.

Unfortunately, fruits and vegetables are largely evaluated by wholesalers and retailers in terms of size, color, shape, texture and pest damage. One would think the most obvious measurement of quality, taste, would be included in such a classification. However, wholesalers and retailers feel taste is unimportant and it isn't evaluated.[67] In short, cosmetic factors are the major criteria.

Due to Federal grades and private grade standards, premium prices go to the most cosmetically perfect produce. To get the best prices, farmers use more pesticides. According to the consumer group, Public Voice for Food and Health Policy, "High cosmetic quality standards, including those in U.S.D.A. grades, are a significant barrier to the reduction of pesticide use in growing fruits and vegetables."[68]

But on a positive note it adds, "The produce marketing industry is likely to accept lower cosmetic quality standards as the industry learns that consumers are willing to accept some imperfections in their produce in exchange for lower pesticide usage."[69] In other words, consumers would be more apt to buy less-than-perfect fruits and vegetables if the industry or the Agriculture Department would convince the public that blemished produce means fewer pesticides.

Because greater labor is involved with growing organic fruits and vegetables, organic produce usually cost more than commercially grown produce. Do not let the high prices discourage you. Spending more for organic food is a worthwhile investment. It is certainly better to have bigger produce bills than it is to face enormous hospital bills. Commercially grown foods (foods that are bursting with contaminants) may cause cancers, birth defects, nervous disorders, and other illnesses. On the other hand, organically grown foods may not cause such health problems.

According to a Louis Harris poll conducted for *Organic Gardening* magazine, (the leading publication for organic food growers) 84 percent of 1,250 randomly selected adults said that they would purchase organically grown produce if it cost the same as regular (commercially grown) produce.[70] This survey also revealed that 50 percent of the 1,250 respondents said that they were willing to pay more for organic food.[71] As demands grow and the nation goes "organic," consumers can expect to see lower prices.

If your produce store and supermarket only carry a limited selection of organically grown food, or do not carry any at all, tell the produce manager that there is a big demand for such food. You may also want to consider purchasing organically grown food by mail. See Appendix 1 for a list of more than 100 organic mail-order food suppliers. Many of these suppliers offer competitive prices.

NOTES

CHAPTER 1.
FIGHTING PESTICIDES, INSECTICIDES, AND OTHER TOXIC CHEMICALS IN OUR FOOD SUPPLY

1. Keith Schneider, "Fears of Pesticides Threaten American Way of Farming." *The New York Times*, May 1, 1989, p. Al.

2. Figures released in March 1989, by Janet Hathaway, Senior Lobbyist for Natural Resources Defense Council (NRDC), and Robin Wyatt, Senior Project Scientist for NRDC.

3-4. James C. McCullagh, "A Mother's Crusade." *Organic Gardening*, April 1989, p. 32.

5. *Organic Gardening*, April 1989, p. 34.

6-7. Philip Shabecoff, "Apple Sales Rise After Scare of '89." *The New York Times*, November 13, 1990, p. A28.

8. Marian Burros, "Hazards on the Table: Fears Rise Over Safety of Food Supply." *The New York Times*, May 7, 1990, p. Dll.

9. Keith Schneider, "Curbs on Deadly Insecticide Are Urged." *The New York Times*, March 21, 1989 and *The New York Times*, May 7, 1990, p. Dll.

10-11. *The New York Times*, March 21, 1989.

12-17. *The New York Times*, May 7, 1990, p. Dll.

18-20. *The New York Times*, May 1, 1989, p. A14.

21. Debra Lynn Dadd, *The Nontoxic Home* (Los Angeles: Tarcher, 1986), p. 121.

22. *The Nontoxic Home*, p. 122.

23. *The Nontoxic Home*, p. 123.

24-30. Marlise Simmons, "Concern Rising Over Harm From Pesticides in Third World." *The New York Times*, May 30, 1989, p. C4.

31. *The New York Times*, May 7, 1990, p. Dll.

32. Marian Burros, "Good Health Habits Can Reduce Risks Of Hazards in Food." *The New York Times*, May 9, 1990, pp. C1, C4.

33-34. *The New York Times*, May 7, 1990, p. Al.

35. *The Nontoxic Home*, p. 127.

36. *The Animals' Voice Magazine*, February 1989, p. 63.

37-38. *The Nontoxic Home*, p. 127.

39-40. *The Animals' Voice Magazine*, February 1989, p. 63.

41-43. Facts presented by Dr. Michael Klaper at the Vegetarian Conference in Dolgeville, NY, August 1988.

44. Nathaniel Mead, "Meat Defeat: Europeans Say No to U.S. Growth Hormones." *EastWest*, May 1990, p. 40.

45-46. Facts presented by Dr. Michael Klaper at the Vegetarian Conference in Dolgeville, NY, August 1988.

47-49. Jane E. Brody, "Personal Health: Safety Questions About Eating Fish." *The New York Times*, June 12, 1991, p. C10.

50-53. Henry Miller, "Chemicals Can Find Their Way Into Dinner." *USA Today*, May 23, 1991, p. 9C.

54-55. *The Nontoxic Home*, p. 127.

56. *The Nontoxic Home*, p. 129.

57-62. *Health Science*, March/April 1989, p. 7.

63. Keith Schneider, "Science Academy Recommends Resumption of Natural Farming: Subsidies Found to Encourage Chemical Overuse." *The New York Times*, September 8, 1989, p. A1.

64-65. *The New York Times*, September 8, 1989, p. B5.

66-69. Marian Burros, "Eating Well: That Blemished Produce May Be the Most Healthful to Eat." *The New York Times*, April 3, 1991, p. C3.

70-71. Joanna Poncavage, "Sold On Organic." *Organic Gardening*, June 1989, p. 43.

2

THE ROAD TO A TOXIC-FREE BODY BEGINS WITH HEALTHY LIVING

Sylvester Graham, the inventor of the popular cracker that bears his name, is often credited as America's first crusader for healthful living. In the early nineteenth century, Graham introduced the healthy lifestyle known as Natural Hygiene. Natural Hygiene emphasizes the remarkable benefits of a diet rich in fresh fruits and vegetables. Natural Hygiene also recognizes the importance of clean air, bathing, exercise, rest and relaxation, and mental stimulation.

Although Graham's principles for a healthy lifestyle may not seem unusual, it must be pointed out that just over a century ago many of his principles were considered by most physicians as revolutionary and radical.[1] In the 1830's, when Graham introduced his wholesome diet, the medical establishment persisted in denying the health advantages of such a diet. Because of medical ignorance, Graham was harassed throughout his lifetime by physicians for his statements on the health benefits of fruits and vegetables.[2]

Graham was also harassed by physicians for his statements on the need for fresh air. It is interesting to note that the medical value of fresh air is a modern discovery.[3] In the 19th century, fresh air was viewed by many as "infectious" and physicians as well as laymen avoided it as much as possible.[4] According to an article in *The Herald of Health* (London), Feb. 1911, "In early Victorian times the first thing the doctor did when he had a sick patient was to close the windows."[5] Right here in the United States in the 1800's, medical doctors claimed the air of the cities was more suitable for asthmatics than that of the country.[6] Such doctors insisted the more polluted the air, the better it was for people suffering from asthma.[7] In the 1800's, it was not uncommon for physicians to treat asthma by telling patients to breathe fumes from coal-gas factories.[8]

Graham's views on the health benefits of bathing were also attacked by physicians. The medical establishment in the U.S. in the 1800's considered bathing harmful.[9] According to an article entitled "The Abuses of Bathing" which appeared in the *Boston Medical and Surgical Journal* in 1850, "In our opinion, once a week is often enough to bathe the whole body for purposes of luxury and cleanliness. Beyond this we consider bathing to be injurious."[10]

Graham developed the Natural Hygiene lifestyle in part as a reaction to this medical ignorance. Considering the medical beliefs of that era, Graham proved to have been years ahead of his time.

Other notable health figures of the 19th century include the following medical doctors: John Tilden, Russell Thacker Trall, Isaac Jennings, James Caleb Jackson, Robert Walter, Mary Dodd, and William Hay. These physicians recognized the medical values of Graham's ideas and took up his mission. These doctors played an important role in educating Americans on the advantages of a Natural Hygiene lifestyle.

The above physicians also deserve much credit for exposing the dangers of drugs. These doctors made Americans aware of the fact that if they follow a healthy lifestyle, they will not have to resort to medications or drugs. Dr. James Caleb Jackson was so against medications he felt compelled to write a book about his beliefs. His book, published in 1873, was entitled *How to Treat the Sick Without Medicine.*

Despite relentless criticism from the medical establishment, these Natural Hygiene crusaders spoke their minds and furthered the cause for healthful living. In effect, Natural Hygiene became the forerunner of modern day preventive medicine.

Dr. Herbert M. Shelton became accepted as the Natural Hygiene leader of the 20th century. Towards the end of Shelton's lifetime (1895-1985), the Natural Hygiene movement achieved world-wide recognition and respect. Shelton founded in 1928 the first Natural Hygiene Health School in San Antonio, Texas. He was also the author of over forty books which promote the Natural Hygiene lifestyle.

Shelton advanced the Natural Hygiene lifestyle by introducing an eating plan that prevents indigestion and heartburn. By observing thousands of patients, Shelton discovered this eating plan which he referred to as "food combining principles." Shelton said, "The haphazard and indiscriminate jumbling together at the same meal of foods of all kinds...result in much indigestion and discomfort."[11] By following correct food combinations, never again will you need Alka-Seltzer, Rolaids, Tums, or any other antacid formula.

In order to prevent indigestion and heartburn, you are advised to keep meals simple. Shelton believed that digestion of food is best accomplished if only one kind of food is eaten at a time. For instance, melons should be eaten alone as a meal, without any other food. Shelton found that different foods require different time periods to digest. He maintained that food not digested quickly and efficiently leads to a buildup of toxins in the digestive tract. Shelton claimed that degenerative diseases result from accumulation of toxins not eliminated.

Food Combining Principles For Preventing Indigestion:

Most fruits may be eaten with most other fruits.

Melons should be eaten alone. Melons should make up the meal.

Proteins should not be eaten with carbohydrates in the same meal. Fats should not be eaten with proteins in the same meal.

Most vegetables may be eaten with proteins or carbohydrates in the same meal.

The Natural Hygiene Diet is only part of the total Hygienic way of LIFE. Some basic principles of Natural Hygiene in addition to eating healthful foods, include the need for a toxic-free surrounding, exercise, rest and relaxation, and mental stimulation. Each element of Natural Hygiene is as important as the other.[12]

Although one may think it is too much of a burden and too costly to create a toxic-free surrounding, this is hardly the case. Procedures for creating a toxic-free surrounding are remarkably simple and inexpensive. To start with, see to it that you receive as much clean air as possible. Your home as well as the workplace should be well ventilated. Also, don't smoke. More than 400,000 Americans die from breathing their own smoke each year.[13]

The lungs are not the only organs that are heavily damaged by cigarette smoke. Other parts of the body are also seriously injured by cigarette smoke. New studies show that smoking causes damage to the brain and heart, among other effects. These findings place stroke and heart disease on the list with lung cancer as deadly illnesses linked to smoking.

Researchers found that cigarette smoke impairs the arteries that supply the brain and increases the risk of one kind of stroke. Researchers discovered that a 50-year-old person who is a heavy smoker (a person who smokes two packs of cigarettes a day) has artery damage comparable to a light smoker who is 60 years old.[14] According to Dr. Robert Dempsey, a neurosurgeon at the University of Kentucky, "The effect in that 50-year-old would be to take 10 years off his life."[15]

Another study found that people who smoked a pack a day or less were four times as likely as nonsmokers to suffer from a deadly form of stroke called subarachnoid hemorrhage.[16] This stroke occurs most often in people under 65 and it is more common in women. Subarachnoid hemorrhages account for 7 percent of the 500,000 strokes suffered by Americans each year.[17]

It has been shown that those who smoked more than a pack a day had up to 11 times the risk of developing subarachnoid hemorrhages.[18] Dr. Will Longstreth, a neurologist at the University of Washington, claimed the risk of suffering a subarachnoid hemorrhage is especially high within three hours of smoking a cigarette, and then drops off gradually.[19] Dr. Longstreth concluded that smoking was responsible for almost 38 percent of all subarachnoid hemorrhages.[20] He said that more than 8,000 of those strokes could be prevented each year in the United States if people stopped smoking.[21]

Do not believe those who claim that second-hand smoke is not harmful. Tobacco smoke is the number one toxic pollutant humans are most often exposed to. Be prudent and keep away from those who smoke. And see to it that "no-smoking" laws are strictly enforced. Daily exposure to second-hand smoke can needlessly hasten one's death. By regularly staying in places where people smoke, one is greatly jeopardizing one's life. Second-hand smoke causes thousands of deaths to nonsmokers each year.

Recent studies confirm that second-hand smoke or sidestream smoke as it is commonly called, is extremely dangerous. New findings reveal that the damage done by sidestream smoke is not just limited to the lungs. Sidestream smoke has been proven to cause damage to the blood vessels and heart.[22] Research has shown that the toxic fumes produced by smokers can cause heart damage in people who breathe them.[23] Doctors have found a strong link between sidestream smoke and heart disease. The carbon monoxide in cigarette smoke impairs red blood cells in carrying oxygen throughout the body, forcing the heart to work harder.

Other chemicals in second-hand smoke injures cells in the lining of arteries, encouraging the formation of fatty plaques. Second-hand smoke also makes clot-forming platelets stickier, encouraging them to clot on the plaques and promoting arteriosclerosis, the primary cause of most heart attacks.[24] Dr. Stanton A.

Glantz, a cardiologist researcher at the University of California at San Francisco, estimated that sidestream smoke killed 50,000 Americans a year, two-thirds of whom died of heart disease.[25]

Dr. Glantz estimated that one-third of the 50,000 deaths from sidestream smoke were from cancer.[26] Sidestream smoke has been linked to cancers of the brain, thyroid, and breast.[27] According to the EPA, cigarette smoke consists of more than 4,700 compounds, including 43 carcinogens.[28] Dr. Glantz maintained that second-hand smoke ranks behind direct smoking and alcohol as the third leading preventable cause of death in the United States.[29]

There are other, often overlooked, methods for creating a cleaner, safer environment. Such methods are also simple and inexpensive. By lowering the use of harmful chemical cleaners, polishes, aerosol sprays, bug sprays, paint thinners, and solvents, you are contributing greatly to a toxic-free surrounding.

Chemical air fresheners do not have to be used to get rid of household odors. Manufacturers of air fresheners want us to believe that their products are the only solution to an unpleasant smell. In their attempt to win us over, manufacturers of air fresheners like to link their products to nature and the environment. For example, television commercials portray housewives who praise and stress the "naturalness" of air fresheners. They may say the air freshener has a "fresh lemon scent" or the air freshener "brings the scent of a pine forest into your home."

What the makers of air fresheners do not tell us in their television commercials or other advertisements is that the fresh lemon scent or pine forest scent is made from harmful synthetic fragrances. All these products do is temporarily mask an odor with poisonous fragrances. Thus, they are in effect adding more pollutants. The safest and most effective air freshener is an opened window.

Chemical carpet cleaners and carpet fresheners are harmful and unnecessary. Chemical carpet cleaners and carpet fresheners are in the same category with air fresheners. Manufacturers of carpet cleaners/fresheners also like to link their products to nature and the environment. Television commercials and other advertisements claim the carpet cleaner/freshener "removes odors and leaves your carpet smelling like fresh flowers," or the carpet cleaner/freshener "removes odors and leaves your carpet with a fresh country scent."

Why do the makers of air fresheners and carpet cleaners/fresheners use references to nature and the environment to sell their products? The answer is very simple: It is a scheme to disguise and cover-up the harmful contents of these products, and to trick the consumer into thinking these products are perfectly safe.

Another reason why manufacturers link their products to nature and the environment is because it's the "in" thing to do. Due to an increased awareness and a renewed interest in the environment, the environment has become a very "hot" selling device. Since everybody wants to "cash in" on the environment, it comes as no surprise that manufacturers of air fresheners and carpet cleaners/fresheners use the environment as part of their sales pitch.

Chemical carpet cleaners/fresheners do nothing more than add artificial fragrances and poisons to your home. The safest and most effective carpet cleaner/freshener is baking soda. That's right, plain old baking soda (the kind used for baking).

Make sure the carpet is dry before pouring on the baking soda. Sprinkle it generously (it is cheap enough). Wait one hour or longer, then vacuum. For stubborn odors, sprinkle greater amounts of baking soda and leave it on the carpet overnight. Vacuum it the next day. Here again we see that the safest and the best are also the least expensive.

In his writings, Shelton emphasized the importance of fresh air. According to Shelton, fresh air is necessary for every function of the body.[30] Shelton wrote, "If we prefer the dust-and-poison-laden air of the city to the fresh air of the country, we cannot expect to maintain vigorous health."[31] He added, "The elasticity and cheerfulness of perfect health can never be experienced in a life habitually passed indoors."[32]

Exercise is a key element of Natural Hygiene. Shelton said, "Extensive experience has shown that inaction diminishes the size of a bone, injures its structure and deprives it of hardness to such an extent that it may be cut with a knife. Bones subjected to strenuous use became harder, tougher, larger, and less liable to injury."[33]

Before choosing an exercise or sport make sure it is suitable for your physical condition. If for example, you suffer from lower back pain, tennis or jogging may be very painful activities. And since these activities may even exacerbate your condition it is important to avoid participating in them. Do not feel badly. There are alternatives. For instance, swimming may be an ideal form of exercise for those who suffer from back pain. If you are unsure whether an exercise or sport is appropriate for you, it is best to check with your physician.

It is also best to choose an exercise program or sport that you enjoy participating in. This way you'll be less likely to get bored or lose motivation.

As a wonderful bonus, exercise may put you in a great state of mind and may really make you feel good. What causes this sensation? And how does it occur? The clues to these questions are to be found in a chemical produced by the body. When you exercise, the body manufactures chemicals known as endorphins (morphine-like substances) which give the effect of a natural-high. Though participants of any sport may experience a natural-high, this phenomenon is especially pronounced among runners and joggers. Endorphins might help explain why running, jogging, and other sports may be addictive.

Rest and relaxation are central to Natural Hygiene. Proper rest and sleep are signs of good health. If necessary, take a rest in the middle of the day or an afternoon nap to alleviate fatigue and maintain well-being.

Mental stimulation is also an important element of Natural Hygiene. Natural Hygiene teaches us to constantly engage in mental expression. Shelton remarked, "A brain that is not used deteriorates in the same manner as unused muscles."[34]

To sum it up, the Natural Hygiene lifestyle can be a safe, effective regimen for everyone-including infants, adolescents, pregnant women, and the elderly.

NOTES

CHAPTER 2.
THE ROAD TO A TOXIC-FREE BODY BEGINS WITH HEALTHY LIVING

1-2. Herbert M. Shelton, *The Hygienic System Vol.II* (San Antonio: Dr. Shelton's Health School, 1956), p. 10.

3. Herbert M. Shelton, *Health For The Millions* (Chicago: Natural Hygiene Press, 1968), p. 217.

4-7. *Health For The Millions*, p. 216.

8. *Health For The Millions*, p. 217.

9-10. Harvey and Marilyn Diamond, *Living Health* (New York: Warner, 1987), p. 198.

11. Jean A. Oswald, *Yours For Health: The Life and Times of Herbert M. Shelton* (Franklin, Wisconsin: Franklin Books, 1989), p. 67.

12. *Yours For Health*, p. 124.

13. "Death Toll From Smoking Is Worsening." *The New York Times*, February 1, 1991, p. A14.

14-21. "Two Studies Disclose Dangers To Brain Caused by Smoking." *The New York Times*, February 25, 1991, p. A6.

22-25. Lawerence K. Altman, "The Evidence Mounts On Passive Smoking." *The New York Times*, May 29, 1990, p. C1.

26-29. *The New York Times*, May 29, 1990, p. C8. Jane E. Brody, "New Study Strongly Links Passive Smoking and Cancer." *The New York Times*, January 8, 1992, p. C12.

30-32. *Health For The Millions*, p. 220.

33. *Health For The Millions*, p. 242.

34. *Health For The Millions*, p. 283.

3

HOW TO PREVENT TOXEMIA

When toxins are not eliminated from the body, one has the condition known as Toxemia. Toxemia results when the bloodstream and tissues become saturated with toxins. We poison ourselves in two ways: from within the body (Endogenous Toxemia) and from what we take into the body from the outside-toxic substances such as tobacco smoke and harmful foods (Exogenous Toxemia).[1]

Chronic or long term Toxemia results in disease. If there is a saturation of toxins and it is not stopped and reversed, Toxemia continues, progressing through seven stages. According to Shelton, "Although not every disease follows each stage, all diseases are an orderly progression from low energy levels to pathological degeneration."[2] Here are the seven stages:

1. Enervation (general weakness). Nerve energy is reduced and normal body functions are impaired, especially the process of elimination.

2. Toxemia. Nerve energy is too low to eliminate metabolic wastes. Because nerve energy is too low to eliminate toxins, the bloodstream and cells become saturated with toxins.

3. Irritation. A toxic buildup within the tissues results in irritability and nausea.

4. Inflammation. Toxins have accumulated and parts of the body become inflamed. Every part of the body when inflamed, give rise to its own symptom-complex, or what is known as a special disease. Shelton said, "The disease can be named because of its location and different tissues involved."[3]

5. Ulceration. Tissues are destroyed during a process in which the body ulcerates and forms an outlet for the toxic buildup.

6. Induration. Ulcerated tissue hardens or scars.

7. Chronic Degeneration. Cellular activity is destroyed through disorganization or proliferation of diseased cells. Death occurs due to the failure of vital organs.

Shelton claimed, "Those who understand this orderly progression into sickness can reverse the process provided an irreversible stage has not been reached."[4]

Drugs and medications, with their toxic side effects, send thousands to hospitals every year with drug-caused illnesses and large numbers of premature deaths.[5] This chapter presents a dietary approach for preventing and treating diseases.

Hypertension

For the prevention and treatment of hypertension (high blood pressure) follow these guidelines:

Go on a low-sodium, low-fat, high-fiber diet.

Avoid eating meat and animal products.

Eat foods rich in fiber. Vegetarians and others who eat high-fiber foods have lower blood pressure levels than those who eat meat and foods with little fiber.[6]

Eat foods rich in potassium such as fruits and vegetables.

Consume small amounts of vegetable oils. Polyunsaturated vegetable fats tend to lower blood pressure.[7]

Reduce your intake of alcoholic beverages. Some scientists claim alcohol may cause the arterioles to constrict.[8]

Limit your intake of caffeinated beverages. Two or three cups of coffee a day can raise both the systolic and diastolic pressure of a normal person.[9] (By avoiding caffeine, you are significantly lowering the risks of developing numerous diseases. Caffeine has been linked to birth defects in animals. Caffeine is suspected of causing birth defects in humans.[10] Cancer of the urinary bladder also has been linked to caffeine use.)[11]

Avoid taking over-the-counter drugs containing caffeine. Caffeine may be present in analgesics, diuretics, and stimulants.

Avoid taking over-the-counter drugs containing phenylpropanolamine (also known as PPA). PPA is found in various cold, allergy, and diet medications.[12]

Avoid taking other medications that increase blood pressure.

Try to avoid stressful situations.

Try to maintain your ideal weight.

Exercise daily.

Atherosclerosis and Heart Disease

Follow these guidelines to lower your risk of developing atherosclerosis and heart disease. Those already diagnosed with atherosclerosis or heart disease may also benefit.

Cut down your intake of all animal products. Cholesterol is the main cause of atherosclerosis-hardening of the arteries. (Cholesterol is found only in animal foods.)

Go on a low-fat, high-fiber diet. Eat fruits and vegetables rich in fiber.[13]

Eat foods rich in beta carotene such as carrots, cantaloupe, sweet potatoes, broccoli, and kale.[14]

If you have a high cholesterol level, discontinue the practice of drinking coffee. Coffee may increase the rate of atherosclerosis.[15] Caffeine is a known cardiac toxin. Also bear in mind, coffee contains numerous chemical substances, most of which have not been evaluated for safety. From a nutritional standpoint, coffee has no redeeming value.

Increase your intake of vitamin B3 (niacin). Vitamin B3 has been shown to reduce cholesterol levels. Foods rich in vitamin B3 include whole grains, nuts, and beans.[16]

Eat raw cucumbers. Studies have shown that sterols from cucumbers help the body excrete cholesterol.[17]

Eat a lot of citrus fruits. Citrus fruits contain terpenes, natural compounds that limit the synthesis of cholesterol in the body.[18]

Eat fresh garlic. Fresh garlic contains sulfur compounds that have been proven to lower blood pressure and reduce cholesterol.[19]

Consume small amounts of polyunsaturated fats such as vegetable oils. Polyunsaturated fats tend to lower blood pressure.[20]

If you are a hostile person and have an angry disposition look for ways to become more cheerful. Chronic anger (getting upset over anything and everything) is a serious health hazard. Researchers found that hostile people are more likely than others to have a reactive sympathetic nervous system. Their bodies often produce abnormally high levels of stress hormones such as adrenaline and noradrenaline whenever they feel that somebody is picking on them. These stress hormones produced by the sympathetic nervous system raise blood pressure and heart rate, among other effects.[21]

In the chronically hostile, the parasympathetic nervous system does not function well. The parasympathetic nervous system manufactures the common hormone acetylcholine which is responsible for neutralizing the harsh effects of adrenaline. Over a period, too much adrenaline and too little acetylcholine can wreak havoc. The arteries become stiffened from a constantly elevated blood pressure and the heart becomes weak from being overexerted. Recent studies also show that stress hormones damage the liver and kidney.[22] It has also been found that stress hormones release too much fat from fat storage areas of the body into the bloodstream. This action might explain why those who are hostile as teen-agers have high cholesterol levels as adults.[23]

Exercise daily.

Cancer

Although the technique of "fasting" (see Chapter 5) as advanced by Dr. Herbert M. Shelton, is the best method for eliminating toxins from the body, it is not a treatment for cancer. Shelton said, "I have seen cancerous growths greatly reduce in size during a fast, but I have never seen one totally eliminated. And in some cases, cancerous tumors persist in growing, even through a long fast. Only benign tumors frequently disappear after the fast. Fasting does not remedy cancer, and I am convinced that it may hasten death in cancer of the pancreas and of the liver. In other types of cancer its tendency is to prolong life and lessen suffering."[24]

Following these guidelines may prevent several forms of cancers, especially cancer of the colon, a common and deadly form of cancer. Colon cancer ranks behind lung cancer as the second most prevalent form of cancer in the United States.[25]

Go on a low-cholesterol, low-fat, low-sodium, high-fiber diet. It has been proven that the more red meat and animal fat that people eat, the more likely they are to develop colon cancer.[26]

Eat fruits and vegetables rich in vitamin A (beta carotene) and vitamin C. A diet deficient in vitamin A has been linked to cancers of the prostate gland, cervix, skin, bladder, and colon.[27]

Eat cruciferous vegetables such as cabbage, broccoli, Brussels sprouts, kohlrabi, and cauliflower.

Eat foods rich in indoles. Indoles are found in vegetables of the cabbage family (cabbage, broccoli, cauliflower, mustard greens, kale, etc.).[28]

Eat plenty of citrus fruits. Compounds known as terpenes found in citrus fruits such as oranges stimulate enzymes to block the action of carcinogens.[29]

Increase your intake of fresh parsley. Parsley contains polyacetylenes, natural agents that block the synthesis of prostaglandins that promote cancer. Polyacetylenes also suppress the carcinogen benzopyrene (a lethal hydrocarbon found in cigarette smoke).[30]

Eat fresh garlic often. Sulfur compounds in fresh garlic intercept cancer-causing substances and retard tumor development. Garlic even has the effect of encouraging precancerous cells to return to their normal state.[31]

Eat legumes (peanuts, peas and beans). Compounds known as isoflavones found in legumes have been shown to inactivate cancer gene enzymes.[32]

Avoid meats containing nitrites. Such meats include ham, hot dogs, sausage, cold cuts, and bacon. (If you are unable to give up eating meat, switch to organically raised beef.)

Avoid foods containing hydrogenated or partially hydrogenated vegetable oils. Such foods include margarine, vegetable shortening, and imitation milk.

Avoid foods containing artificial preservatives, flavorings, and colorings.

As suspected carcinogens, avoid these artificial sweeteners: saccharin, cyclamate, and aspartame.

Avoid highly salted vegetables such as pickles and other highly salted foods. Such foods may cause stomach cancer.[33] Due to a diet high in salt, the Japanese have one of the highest rates of stomach cancer in the world.[34]

Don't eat charcoal-broiled or any smoked foods. When foods are charcoal-broiled or smoked, carcinogens are formed.

Avoid talc-coated rice (contains asbestos). Talc-coated rice may cause stomach cancer and other cancers of the gastrointestinal tract.[35]

Limit your intake of alcoholic beverages. Heavy consumption of alcohol may cause cancers of the mouth, throat, esophagus, and liver. [36] (By avoiding alcoholic beverages you are preventing serious damage to the liver, one of the major organs that removes toxins from the body.)

Kidney Disease

To prevent and treat most kidney diseases and most kinds of kidney stones, follow these guidelines:

To stop or slow down most kinds of kidney failure it is necessary to go on a low-protein, low-fat, low-sodium, no-cholesterol, high-fiber diet. [37]

Eat mostly starch foods such as potatoes, sweet potatoes, corn, rice, and other whole grains.

Eliminate foods that cause allergic reactions.

People who have advanced kidney failure, those with less than 25 percent kidney function, or patients on dialysis should eat mostly grains such as rice, and fruits and vegetables low in potassium. A low-potassium diet is essential to prevent the buildup of dangerous levels of potassium in the blood. Patients with less than 25 percent kidney function should be under a doctor's supervision and receive frequent blood tests to ensure that the bloodstream does not reach dangerous levels of potassium. [38]

Treatments for removing painful kidney stones may call for pulverization (using sophisticated ultrasonic equipment) or surgery. The preferred treatment, aside from a change in diet, is the pulverization procedure.

Ulcers

Follow these guidelines for relief of painful ulcers:

Avoid drinking caffeinated beverages.

Avoid drinking carbonated drinks.

Avoid drinking beer.

Avoid drinking tea.

Avoid drinking coffee (regular, decaffeinated, and acid-neutralized).

Avoid drinking milk. Milk offers only temporary relief. Milk has a "rebound" effect. After a certain amount of acid has been buffered, the calcium and protein in milk stimulate the production of even more acid.[39]

Eat several meals throughout the day. Don't keep your stomach empty for a long period. By eating constantly throughout the day, digestive juices in the stomach will be able to act on food and not on the empty stomach.

Diabetes

To prevent and alleviate all forms of diabetes follow these guidelines:

Go on a no-cholesterol, low-fat, moderate-protein, high-complex carbohydrate, high-fiber diet.

50 to 60 percent of your total caloric intake should consist of carbohydrates.[40]

Avoid glucose and glucose containing disaccharides such as sucrose and lactose.

Avoid alcoholic beverages.

Avoid caffeinated beverages.

Attempt to reduce insulin injections and medications under your doctor's supervision.

Engage in daily physical activity.

Arthritis

For preventing and treating all forms of arthritis follow these guidelines:

Go on a low-fat, no-cholesterol, low-protein, low-purine, low-allergen diet.

Avoid foods rich in purines. Purines are some of the essential building blocks of DNA and RNA in proteins. Foods rich in purines are foods high in protein such as red meat, poultry, fish, shellfish, and legumes.[41]

Limit your intake of foods that cause allergic reactions. Be especially cautious of dairy products and eggs.

Your diet should consist mostly of starches such as fresh fruits and vegetables.

Avoid alcoholic beverages.

Osteoporosis

To prevent and treat this bone-crippling disease follow these guidelines:

Go on a low-protein diet.

If you are unable to give up high-protein foods, eat foods rich in calcium such as broccoli and greens or take a calcium supplement in pill or tablet form. Do not use dairy products as a calcium supplement. Consumption of dairy products (which are generally high in saturated fat and cholesterol) are responsible for various harmful health effects such as heart disease.[42]

Avoid drinking caffeinated beverages.

Avoid drinking alcoholic beverages.

Avoid drinking sodas. All sodas except club soda may contain phosphorus. Phosphorus robs the body of calcium and causes a chemical imbalance in the body.

Exercise daily.

Asthma

For the treatment of asthma follow these guidelines:

Avoid foods that cause allergic reactions. Be cautious of dairy products, eggs, wheat, and corn.

Breathe clean fresh air. Make sure your house or apartment is well ventilated. If possible, avoid living in large polluted cities.

If you have a gas stove replace it with an electric one. Gas stoves emit fumes that might bring on an asthmatic attack or worsen your existing condition.[43]

Avoid strenuous activity.

Avoid stressful situations.

Avoid exposure to the cold.

Depression

To treat mild forms of depression follow these guidelines:

Your diet should consist mostly of complex carbohydrates.

Eat foods rich in B-complex vitamins such as grains, nuts, and seeds.[44]

Eat foods rich in magnesium such as fresh green vegetables, corn, soybeans, and nuts.[45]

Get more sunlight. If you live in the northern latitudes and get depressed during the winter, money spent on a vacation to the Caribbean may be better spent than visiting a psychiatrist.[46]

Exercise. Exercise produces chemicals in the body called endorphins which give the body a natural-high.

A healthy combination of these principles with a hopeful and positive mental attitude should do much to lift most mild forms of depression.

NOTES

CHAPTER 3.
HOW TO PREVENT TOXEMIA

1. Jean A. Oswald, *Yours For Health: The Life and Times of Herbert M. Shelton* (Franklin, Wisconsin: Franklin Books, 1989), p. 34.

2-4. *Yours for Health*, p. 59.

5. Herbert M. Shelton, *Health For The Millions* (Chicago: Natural Hygiene Press, 1968), p. 3.

6. Evelyn Zamula, "Preventing High Blood Pressure." U.S. Department of Health and Human Services, September 1986.

7. John A. McDougall, *McDougall's Medicine* (Piscataway, New Jersey: New Century, 1985), pp. 116, 188.

8-9. Evelyn Zamula, "Preventing High Blood Pressure." U.S. Department of Health and Human Services, September 1986.

10. John A. and Mary A. McDougall, *The McDougall Plan* (Piscataway, New Jersey: New Century, 1983), p. 175.

11. *The McDougall Plan*, p. 176.

12. Evelyn Zamula, "Preventing High Blood Pressure." U.S. Department of Health and Human Services, September 1986.

13. *McDougall's Medicine*, p. 113.

14. Denise Webb, "Eating Well: A Study of the Effects of Beta Carotene." *The New York Times*, November 28, 1990, P. C3.

15. *McDougall's Medicine*, p. 114.

16. *McDougall's Medicine*, p. 115.

17-19. Jane E. Brody, "Fortified Foods Could Fight Off Cancer." *The New York Times*, February 19, 1991, pp. Cl, C8.

20. *McDougall's Medicine*, pp. 116, 188.

21-23. Natalie Angier, "If Anger Ruins Your Day, It Can Shrink Your Life." *The New York Times*, December 13, 1990, p. B23.

24. *Yours For Health*, p. 121.

25. Gina Kolata, "Animal Fat Is Tied to Colon Cancer: Largest Study of Diet in U.S. Backs Long-Held Theory." *The New York Times*, December 13, 1990, pp. A1, B20.

26. *The New York Times*, December 13, 1990, pp. Al, B20.

27. "Diet Nutrition and Cancer Prevention," National Cancer Institute, December 1986 and *The New York Times*, November 28, 1990, p. C3.

28-32. *The New York Times*, February 19, 1991, pp. Cl, C8. Janice M. Horowitz, "Wonders of the Vegetable Bin." *Time*, September 2, 1991, p. 66.

33-34. *The McDougall Plan*, p. 150.

35. *The McDougall Plan*, p. 148.

36. *The McDougall Plan*, p. 175.

37. *McDougall's Medicine*, p. 271.

38. *McDougall's Medicine*, pp. 269, 271.

39. Louise Fenner, "When Digestive Juices Corrode, You've Got An Ulcer." U.S. Department of Health and Human Services, July/August 1984.

40. "Principles of Nutrition and Dietary Recommendations for Individuals with Diabetes Mellitus: 1979," *Journal of the American Dietetic Association*, 75: 527-530.

41. *McDougall's Medicine*, p. 234.

42. *McDougall's Medicine*, p. 89.

43. Debra Lynn Dadd, *The Nontoxic Home* (Los Angeles: Tarcher, 1986), p. 171.
Alfred V. Zamm and Robert Gannon, *Why Your House May Endanger Your Health* (New York: Simon and Shuster, 1980), pp. 54-55.

44. H.L. Newbold, *Mega-Nutrients For Your Nerves* (New York: Berkley Books, 1981, paperback edition), pp. 130, 133.

45. Earl Mindell, *Vitamin Bible* (New York: Warner, 1985), p. 94.

46. *Mega-Nutrients For Your Nerves*, p. 253.

4

A 6-WEEK EATING PLAN FOR A TOXIC-FREE BODY

This chapter focuses on eating guidelines used to achieve a toxic-free body. According to Shelton, fruits are the healthiest foods. He claimed that fruits, especially oranges, grapefruit, tomatoes (botanically speaking, tomatoes are classified as fruits, not vegetables), grapes, and apples, are the best foods that cleanse the body of toxins.[1] Shelton stated, "These fruits are rich in organic salts, which are liberated during digestion, and supply the body with the elements necessary to the neutralization and chemicalization of the toxins preparatory to their elimination."[2]

Although fresh is best, frozen fruits and vegetables that do not contain additives such as sugar or salt, may be eaten when fresh varieties are not available (out of season). Avoid canned fruits and vegetables that contain bad ingredients such as sugar, salt, artificial colorings and flavorings, and harmful preservatives. Canned fruits and vegetables that do not contain additives, and are in lead-free cans, are acceptable.

Even though fruits and vegetables are the most healthful foods, avoid eating cranberries and rhubarb. Cranberries and rhubarb may be considered toxic because they are high in oxalic acid. Oxalic acid chelates calcium from the intestines. In addition, those who eat foods rich in oxalic acid may suffer from nausea, fatigue, and overall weakness.[3]

List of Recommended Foods (Increase Your Intake of These Foods)

Fruits, especially oranges, grapefruit, tomatoes, grapes, and apples

Vegetables

Whole grains

Beans and legumes

Nuts and seeds (unsalted nuts and seeds make great snacks)

A Six-Week Menu

This very tempting and delicious menu is not rigid with regards to quantities. Serving portions are not restricted. You are advised to eat until you are satisfied. If certain foods are not available, they may be replaced with similar ones. Try not to substitute those fruits that are best for eliminating toxins from the body: oranges, grapefruit, tomatoes, grapes, and apples.

The scrumptious salad featured on the menu may consist of sliced tomatoes, sweet red or green peppers, carrots, celery, cucumbers, avocados, lettuce and/or cabbage, and diced onions. You may omit some (though try not to omit tomatoes), or you may add vegetables that suit your taste. For that extra zest, you may sprinkle sunflower seeds or sesame seeds on top of the salad, or add a teaspoon or two of vegetable oil of your choice. For an exquisite taste, add a few cloves of minced garlic topped off with the juice of a freshly squeezed lemon or lime. This scrumptious salad is a major component of the menu; it is meant to be eaten often.

Before rushing to the kitchen to try this mouth-watering menu please be aware of the following information. You don't want to prepare that luscious, healthy dish, only to find out later that the utensils used added toxic substances to your meal.

Avoid using aluminum and copper cookware. Aluminum and copper utensils should not be used for cooking because they react chemically with foods when heated. Toxic chemicals are formed when food is heated in aluminum and copper cookware. High levels of aluminum or copper are released into the food being heated. Although a small amount of copper is safe, a large amount, such as that resulting from foods being cooked in copper pots, can cause nausea, vomiting, insomnia, hair loss, and depression.[4] Foods cooked in aluminum should not be consumed. Aluminum is recognized as a toxic metal; it has been implicated in the development of brain disorders such as Alzheimer's disease.[5]

For health measures, use glass, iron, stainless steel, or enamel as cookware. Though less desirable, brass and monel utensils may be used.

For a toxic-free body, this menu should be followed for six weeks. Those who get hungry between meals may eat nutritious snacks, and should be aware that fresh fruits, dried fruits, and nuts and seeds are convenient, great tasting, wholesome snacks. Choose nuts and seeds that have not been roasted in oil and do not contain salt. Dried fruits should not contain sulfites or other additives. Health food stores are good sources for dried fruits, nuts and seeds, and nut butters.

Pure water (distilled water) is the best liquid to quench a thirst. You may drink water whenever you are thirsty.

When pita bread or whole grain bread is featured on the menu, it is the whole wheat variety. Health food stores are also good places to find whole grain breads, whole wheat spaghetti and macaroni products, and whole wheat pretzels.

Preparations for foods denoted with asterisks (*)
are described at the end of the menu.

1st Week

Sunday

BREAKFAST   LUNCH   DINNER

Grapefruit   *Tasty Pita Sandwich*   *Scrumptious Vegetable Salad*
Oranges   *Healthy Dressing*   *Adzuki Rice Delight*
              Great Tasting Baked Potatoes   Sliced Apples Sprinkled
              Steamed Cauliflower   With Hulled Sesame Seeds

Monday

BREAKFAST   LUNCH   DINNER

Apples   *Delectable Avocado Sandwich*   *Crispy Green Salad*
Peaches   *Hearty Lentil Stew*   *Healthy Dressing*
Bananas   *Chickpea Savory*   Baked Sweet Potatoes
              Filberts   *Tempting Strawberry Dessert*

Tuesday

BREAKFAST   LUNCH   DINNER

Grapes   *Zesty Peanut Butter Sandwich*   *Scrumptious Vegetable Salad*
Cherries   Sunflower Seeds   *Fantastic Split Pea Soup*
Kiwi fruit   Pumpkin Seeds   Brazil Nuts
                                                Pecans
                                                Peanuts

Wednesday

BREAKFAST   LUNCH   DINNER

*Tropical   *Vegetable Ambrosia*   *Scrumptious Vegetable Salad*
  Fruit Juice* *Easy Rice*   *Healthy Dressing*
                Guilt-Free Blueberry Pie   *Delicious Corn*
                                                         Peanuts

Thursday

BREAKFAST   LUNCH   DINNER

Watermelon   *Scrumptious Vegetable Salad*   *Great Tasting Baked Potatoes*
                Healthy Dressing   Steamed String Beans
                Barley Mushroom Soup   Steamed Artichokes
                Walnuts   Steamed Okra

Friday

BREAKFAST   LUNCH   DINNER

Peaches   *Exquisite Vegetable Stew*   *Delectable Avocado Sandwich*
Plums   *Apple Nut A La Mode*   Pistachio Nuts
Bananas   Filberts   Sunflower Seeds

Saturday

BREAKFAST   LUNCH   DINNER

Persimmons   Dried Figs   *Scrumptious Vegetable Salad*
Grapes   Dates   Whole Grain Bread
Apples   Raisins   With Cashew Butter
                Bananas   Almonds

2nd Week

Sunday

BREAKFAST   LUNCH   DINNER

Grapefruit   *Vegetable Cocktail*   *Crispy Green Salad*
Oranges   *Chickpea Savory*   *Healthy Dressing*
                 Pumpkin Seeds   Baked Yams
                                                    Steamed Asparagus

Monday

BREAKFAST   LUNCH   DINNER

Cantaloupe   *Tasty Pita Sandwich*   *Fresh Vegetable Juice*
Honeydew   Steamed Zucchini   *Adzuki Rice Delight*
                 Steamed Okra   *Delicious Corn*
                 Sunflower Seeds   Hulled Sesame Seeds
                                                    (No special preparations are
                                                    needed, just eat right out of
                                                    the package like a snack)

Tuesday

BREAKFAST   LUNCH   DINNER

Apples   *Scrumptious Vegetable Salad*   *Vegetable Ambrosia*
Nectarines   *Gourmet Kasha*   *Crispy Green Salad*
Plums   Filberts   *Great Tasting Baked Potatoes*
                 Walnuts

Wednesday

BREAKFAST   LUNCH   DINNER

Orange Juice   *Hearty Lentil Stew*   *Kidney Bean Supreme*
and/or   Whole Wheat Pretzels   *Easy Rice*
Grapefruit Juice Popcorn (no salt, no oil)   Almonds
                                                    Pecans

Thursday

BREAKFAST	LUNCH	DINNER
Fresh Pineapple	*Fantastic Split Pea Soup* Whole Grain Bread Brazil Nuts Apples	*Scrumptious Vegetable Salad* *Healthy Dressing* Whole Wheat Spaghetti *Natural Tomato Sauce*

Friday

BREAKFAST	LUNCH	DINNER
Strawberries Kiwi fruit Peaches	*Vegetable Cocktail* *Barley Mushroom Soup* Steamed Broccoli	*Scrumptious Vegetable Salad* *Apple Nut A La Mode* Peanuts

Saturday

BREAKFAST	LUNCH	DINNER
Cantaloupe	*Tasty Pita Sandwich* *Luscious Fruit Salad* Avocado	*Crispy Green Salad* Whole Grain Bread With Almond Butter Pumpkin Seeds

3rd Week

Sunday

BREAKFAST	LUNCH	DINNER
Apples Grapes	*Delectable Avocado Sandwich* Whole Wheat Macaroni *Natural Tomato Sauce*	*Gourmet Kasha* Steamed Asparagus Steamed Okra *Frozen Banana-Date Pie*

Monday

BREAKFAST	LUNCH	DINNER
Mangos	*Potato Salad*	*Scrumptious Vegetable Salad*
Cherries	Steamed String Beans	*Hearty Lentil Stew*
Apricots	*Delicious Corn*	Pistachio Nuts

Tuesday

BREAKFAST	LUNCH	DINNER
Tropical Fruit Juice	*Barley Mushroom Soup*	*Tasty Pita Sandwich*
	Walnuts	*Chickpea Savory*
	Pumpkin Seeds	Steamed Artichokes
	Guilt-Free Blueberry Pie	Steamed Squash

Wednesday

BREAKFAST	LUNCH	DINNER
Watermelon	*Exquisite Vegetable Stew*	*Scrumptious Vegetable Salad*
	Steamed Broccoli	*Easy Rice*
	Steamed Okra	*Mixed Beans*
	Almonds	Sunflower Seeds

Thursday

BREAKFAST	LUNCH	DINNER
Grapefruit	*Vegetable Cocktail*	Whole Wheat Macaroni
Oranges	*Crispy Green Salad*	*Natural Tomato Sauce*
	Healthy Dressing	Steamed Sweet Green Peas
	Tangy Compote	Steamed Cauliflower

Friday

BREAKFAST	LUNCH	DINNER
Peaches	*Chunky Potato Soup*	*Scrumptious Vegetable Salad*
Plums	Steamed Asparagus	*Apple Nut A La Mode*
Bananas	Steamed String Beans	Pistachio Nuts
	Steamed Squash	

Saturday

BREAKFAST	LUNCH	DINNER
Cantaloupe	*Tasty Pita Sandwich*	*Scrumptious Vegetable Salad*
Honeydew	Avocado	Whole Grain Bread
	Pistachio Nuts	With Peanut Butter
		Almonds

4th Week

Sunday

BREAKFAST	LUNCH	DINNER
Apples	*Fantastic Split Pea Soup*	*Scrumptious Vegetable Salad*
Pears	*Chickpea Savory*	*Delicious Corn*
Grapes	Filberts	Steamed Broccoli
		Steamed Cauliflower

Monday

BREAKFAST	LUNCH	DINNER
Kiwi fruit	*Crispy Green Salad*	*Scrumptious Vegetable Salad*
Cherries	*Healthy Dressing*	*Kidney Bean Supreme*
Peaches	*Great Tasting Baked Potatoes*	Walnuts

Tuesday

BREAKFAST	LUNCH	DINNER
Blueberries	*Fresh Vegetable Juice*	*Scrumptious Vegetable Salad*
Strawberries	*Luscious Fruit Salad*	*Hearty Lentil Stew*
Tangerines	*Guilt-Free Blueberry Pie*	Peanuts

Wednesday

BREAKFAST	LUNCH	DINNER
Nectarines	*Tasty Pita Sandwich*	*Scrumptious Vegetable Salad*
Apricots	*Gourmet Kasha*	*Barley Mushroom Soup*
Plums	Almonds	Pistachio Nuts

Thursday

BREAKFAST	LUNCH	DINNER
Papayas	*Mixed Beans*	*Crispy Green Salad*
Peaches	Hulled Sesame Seeds	Whole Wheat Spaghetti
	Sunflower Seeds	*Natural Tomato Sauce*

Friday

BREAKFAST	LUNCH	DINNER
Orange Juice	*Delectable Avocado Sandwich*	*Scrumptious Vegetable Salad*
and/or	Baked Sweet Potatoes	*Zesty Peanut Butter Sandwich*
Grapefruit Juice	Steamed Cauliflower	Apples
	Steamed Broccoli	

Saturday

BREAKFAST	LUNCH	DINNER
Watermelon	*Tasty Pita Sandwich*	*Crispy Green Salad*
	Whole Wheat Pretzels	*Apple Nut A La Mode*
	Filberts	Pistachio Nuts

5th Week

Sunday

BREAKFAST	LUNCH	DINNER
Tropical Fruit Juice	*Vegetable Ambrosia* *Delicious Corn* Peanuts	*Chunky Potato Soup* Steamed Artichokes Steamed Sweet Green Peas *Guilt-Free Blueberry Pie*

Monday

BREAKFAST	LUNCH	DINNER
Persimmons Grapes	*Fresh Vegetable Juice* *Luscious Fruit Salad* *Tempting Strawberry Dessert*	*Scrumptious Vegetable Salad* *Fantastic Split Pea Soup* Whole Grain Bread Almonds

Tuesday

BREAKFAST	LUNCH	DINNER
Apples Pears Plums	*Scrumptious Vegetable Salad* *Healthy Dressing* Sunflower Seeds Peaches	*Vegetable Cocktail* Whole Wheat Spaghetti *Natural Tomato Sauce* Steamed Zucchini

Wednesday

BREAKFAST	LUNCH	DINNER
Cantaloupe	Dried Apricots Dried Papaya Raisins Bananas	*Scrumptious Vegetable Salad* *Barley Mushroom Soup* *Gourmet Kasha*

Thursday

BREAKFAST	LUNCH	DINNER
Mangos	Whole Wheat Pretzels	*Crispy Green Salad*
Peaches	Popcorn (no salt, no oil)	*Potato Salad*
	Almonds	Steamed Broccoli
	Peanuts	Steamed String Beans
		Steamed Cauliflower

Friday

BREAKFAST	LUNCH	DINNER
Tangerines	*Vegetable Cocktail*	*Scrumptious Vegetable Salad*
Grapefruit	Whole Wheat Spaghetti	Whole Grain Bread
	Natural Tomato Sauce	With Almond Butter
	Steamed Asparagus	Peanuts

Saturday

BREAKFAST	LUNCH	DINNER
Kiwi fruit	*Luscious Fruit Salad*	*Crispy Green Salad*
Nectarines	*Delectable Avocado Sandwich*	*Apple Nut A La Mode*
Plums	Sunflower Seeds	Brazil Nuts
	Almonds	Pistachio Nuts

6th Week

Sunday

BREAKFAST	LUNCH	DINNER
Bananas	*Fresh Vegetable Juice*	*Scrumptious Vegetable Salad*
Blueberries	*Zesty Peanut Butter Sandwich*	*Hearty Lentil Stew*
	Delicious Corn	Hulled Sesame Seeds

Monday

BREAKFAST	LUNCH	DINNER
Papayas	Dried Figs	*Scrumptious Vegetable Salad*
Apricots	Raisins	*Chickpea Savory*
	Dates	Walnuts
	Bananas	Filberts

Tuesday

BREAKFAST	LUNCH	DINNER
Orange Juice	*Tasty Pita Sandwich*	*Crispy Green Salad*
and/or	Steamed Cauliflower	*Gourmet Kasha*
Grapefruit Juice	Sunflower Seeds	*Mixed Beans*
	Brazil Nuts	Pistachio Nuts

Wednesday

BREAKFAST	LUNCH	DINNER
Honeydew	Whole Grain Bread	*Scrumptious Vegetable Salad*
	With Macadamia Butter	Whole Wheat Macaroni
	Peanuts	*Natural Tomato Sauce*
	Popcorn (no salt, no oil)	Steamed Okra
		Steamed String Beans

Thursday

BREAKFAST	LUNCH	DINNER
Apples	*Vegetable Ambrosia*	*Fantastic Split Pea Soup*
Cherries	*Delicious Corn*	*Adzuki Rice Delight*
Grapes	Steamed Asparagus	Hulled Sesame Seeds
	Steamed Squash	

Friday

BREAKFAST   LUNCH   DINNER

Strawberries   *Barley Mushroom Soup*   *Crispy Green Salad*
Apricots   Steamed Artichokes   Whole Grain Bread
               Steamed Sweet Green Peas   With Cashew Butter
               Frozen Banana-Date Pie   *Apple Nut A La Mode*
                                            Sunflower Seeds

Saturday

BREAKFAST   LUNCH   DINNER

Tangerines   *Luscious Fruit Salad*   *Scrumptious Vegetable Salad*
Oranges   *Delectable Avocado Sandwich* Pumpkin Seeds
Grapefruit   Pistachio Nuts   Almonds
               Pecans   Apples

Preparations For Foods Denoted With Asterisks (*)

TASTY PITA SANDWICH

For pita bread you may either make your own or purchase it already made. If you opt the latter, whole wheat pita bread can be found at health food stores and supermarkets.

Here is the recipe for making your own pita bread, compliments of Bernice and Shirley Davison, Directors of the Health Oasis.

PITA BREAD

    2 packages dry yeast
1 ½ cups warm water
3 ½ to 4 cups whole wheat flour

In a large bowl, blend yeast and water. Let sit 5 minutes or until yeast is dissolved. Stir in 2 cups of flour. Gradually stir in remaining flour until a stiff dough forms.

On a lightly floured board, knead until smooth and elastic. Then place the dough in an oiled bowl, cover and let rise until doubled (1 to 2 hours). Punch dough down and turn on lightly floured board. Divide in 12 parts. Roll each ball into a thin circle, about 5 inches in diameter. Place the flattened rounds on a baking sheet. Let rise 20 to 30 minutes. Rounds will become fluffy. Bake until browned. Cool on rack. Freezes well. To reheat put in 350 degree oven until warm.

SANDWICH

    1 pita bread
1 medium size tomato, diced thinly
1 green bell pepper or sweet red pepper, diced thinly (stem, center, and seeds removed)
1 cucumber, diced thinly
½ avocado, diced thinly
1 small carrot, diced thinly
1 celery stick, diced thinly
    Clump of green or red cabbage, shredded
2 scallions, diced thinly
    Clump of alfalfa sprouts or sprouts of your choice
    Clump of watercress (optional)

Combine everything (except the pita) in a bowl. Slice off edge of pita so that it has a wide opening. Place this strip that was sliced off and put inside bottom of pita. Stuff pita bread with contents from bowl. Pour *Healthy Dressing* on top (if desired) and serve. If salad in bowl is not used up, squeeze fresh lemon or lime on top and store in refrigerator for next time.

HEALTHY DRESSING

¼ cup sesame tahini (available at health food stores)
¼ cup water
½ clove garlic, finely chopped
    Pinch of fresh parsley or dried parsley
½ lemon, freshly squeezed (optional)

Pour the sesame tahini, water, and lemon juice in a blender or food processor. Put garlic and parsley in and then blend until a desired consistency. For a thicker consistency add more tahini, for a thinner consistency add more water.

GREAT TASTING BAKED POTATOES

3 medium size potatoes
2 celery sticks, minced
2 scallions, minced
    Fresh or dried parsley

Cut the potatoes in half and place in oven. When golden brown remove from oven and place on a serving plate. On the plate, add parsley, minced celery and scallions, then serve.

SCRUMPTIOUS VEGETABLE SALAD

4 tomatoes, sliced
3 sweet red or green bell peppers, sliced (stem, center, and seeds removed)
2 carrots, sliced

2 celery sticks, sliced
2 cucumbers, sliced
1 avocado, sliced
½ head of lettuce and/or cabbage, sliced
1 small onion, diced
2 scallions, sliced
   Clump of alfalfa sprouts or similar sprouts (optional)
   Fresh garlic, minced (optional)
   Juice of freshly squeezed lemon or lime

In a salad bowl, mix all of these ingredients together. If desired, pour *Healthy Dressing* on top and serve.

ADZUKI RICE DELIGHT

1 cup adzuki beans (available at health food stores)
1 cup short-grain brown rice (available at health food stores)
2 celery sticks, finely chopped
1 clove garlic, finely chopped

Put adzuki beans in a bowl, add water and soak overnight. The next day when ready to eat, rinse out beans. In a different bowl put rice in and add water. Let rice soak for 5 minutes, then drain the water. Place adzuki beans and rice in a cooking pot and add fresh water. Put chopped celery and garlic in pot. Cook for 20 minutes, then check to see if more water should be added. If no additional water is necessary, continue cooking for 20 minutes and then serve. If more water is necessary, add it and continue cooking for 20 minutes and then serve. (Either way, the total cooking time is 40 minutes.)

DELECTABLE AVOCADO SANDWICH

2 slices of whole grain bread
1 lettuce leaf

½ avocado, sliced
½ cucumber, sliced
1 thin slice of tomato (optional)
1 thin slice of onion (optional)

On one slice of bread, place the lettuce, avocado, cucumber, onion, and tomato. Make a sandwich.

HEARTY LENTIL STEW

1 cup lentils
1 cup barley
2 cups vegetables, diced
Fresh garlic, minced (optional)
Fresh parsley or parsley flakes

Put lentils and barley in a bowl, add water and soak for 3 minutes. Drain water, place lentils and barley in a cooking pot and add fresh water. Place vegetables such as carrots, celery, green bell pepper, onions, cauliflower, and zucchini in pot. For extra taste, add fresh garlic. Cook for 30 to 40 minutes. Add more water if necessary. Serve. Add parsley, if desired.

CHICKPEA SAVORY

1 cup chickpeas (garbanzos)
½ cup celery, finely chopped
½ cup sweet red pepper, finely chopped (stem, center, and seeds removed)
½ cup green bell pepper, finely chopped (stem, center, and seeds removed)
½ clove garlic, minced or garlic powder

Soak a cup of chickpeas overnight. The next day when ready to eat, drain water. Place chickpeas in a cooking pot. Add fresh water and cook for 20 minutes or until chickpeas are tender. Drain water. Add the celery and pepper. Then put in a serving bowl. Add fresh garlic or garlic powder, if desired. Store leftover in refrigerator.

CRISPY GREEN SALAD

3 cucumbers, sliced
3 green bell peppers, sliced (stem, center, and seeds removed)
2 celery sticks, sliced
1 avocado, sliced
2 scallions, sliced
　Clump of romaine lettuce or iceberg lettuce, sliced
　(Note: Since romaine lettuce is a darker green it contains more nutrients than iceberg lettuce.)
　Clump of green cabbage, shredded
　Pinch of fresh parsley
½ lemon or lime, freshly squeezed (optional)

Put all these vegetables in a salad bowl. Add lemon or lime juice on top and then serve. Refrigerate leftover.

TEMPTING STRAWBERRY DESSERT

2 cups strawberries
1 banana (optional)

Put strawberries in food processor or blender. Blend well. Pour contents in a pie dish. Add slices of banana on top. Place in freezer. Keep in freezer until hard. Serve.

ZESTY PEANUT BUTTER SANDWICH

2 slices of whole grain bread
　Peanut butter
1 cucumber, sliced

Clump of romaine or iceberg lettuce
Clump of alfalfa sprouts or similar sprouts

Spread peanut butter on one slice of bread. On top of this slice put the cucumber, lettuce, and sprouts. Then make a sandwich.

FANTASTIC SPLIT PEA SOUP

1 cup green split peas
1 cup barley
½ cup fresh mushrooms, diced
1 celery stick, diced
1 small onion, diced
Fresh parsley or parsley flakes

Rinse split peas and barley. Then put split peas and barley in a cooking pot and add water. Add the mushrooms, celery, and onion to the pot. Cook for 30 minutes. Add more water if necessary. Serve. For extra taste, add parsley.

TROPICAL FRUIT JUICE

1 papaya
1 mango
3 oranges (seedless oranges, if possible)

With a spoon scoop seeds out of papaya. Discard seeds. Slice papaya in thin strips. Remove and discard the peel. Slice mango in thin strips. Remove and discard the peel. Continue slicing the mango until there is no flesh left on the pit. Discard pit. Remove and discard the peel from the 3 oranges. Then slice oranges in thin strips. If there are seeds, discard them. Put thin strips of papaya, mango, and oranges in a juicer and juice. Serve.

VEGETABLE AMBROSIA

2 medium size carrots
1 celery stick
2 medium size beets

Juice everything together and serve.

EASY RICE

1 cup short-grain brown rice
½ cup fresh mushrooms, diced
1 celery stick, diced
1 small onion, diced
1 clove garlic, minced

Soak rice for about 5 minutes. Rinse. Put rice in a cooking dish and add fresh water. Then put mushrooms, celery, onion, and garlic in cooking dish. Cook for 40 minutes or until tender.

GUILT-FREE BLUEBERRY PIE

2 cups blueberries
1 banana (optional)

Put blueberries in food processor or blender. Blend well. Pour contents in a pie dish. Add slices of banana on top. Place in freezer. Keep in freezer until hard. Serve.

DELICIOUS CORN

3 corn
2 celery sticks, diced

1 sweet red or green bell pepper, diced (stem, center, and seeds removed)

1 small onion, diced

Remove husks from corn. Place corn in steamer and steam until tender. On a large plate, slice corn into small kernels. Add the minced celery, pepper, and onion to this plate and serve. A delicious way to eat corn.

BARLEY MUSHROOM SOUP

1 cup barley

½ cup fresh mushrooms, diced

1 green bell pepper, diced (stem, center, and seeds removed)

1 small onion, diced

1 clove garlic, minced

Fresh parsley or parsley flakes

Rinse barley. Place barley in cooking pot and add water. Add the mushrooms, pepper, onion, and garlic. Cook for 30 minutes. Add more water if necessary. Serve. Add a pinch of parsley, if desired.

EXQUISITE VEGETABLE STEW

1 large tomato, sliced

1 celery stick, chopped

1 medium size carrot, chopped

1 sweet red pepper, chopped (stem, center, and seeds removed)

1 green bell pepper, chopped (stem, center, and seeds removed)

Clump of green cabbage, shredded

¼ cup mushrooms, chopped

¼ cup broccoli, chopped

¼ cup cauliflower, chopped

¼ cup zucchini, chopped

¼ cup string beans, chopped

¼ cup sweet green peas
1 medium size onion, sliced
1 clove garlic, minced
  Fresh parsley or parsley flakes

Put everything in a large cooking pot. Add water and cook for 45 minutes or until tender. Add more water if necessary. Serve. Add parsley, if desired.

APPLE NUT A LA MODE

2 large red delicious apples, sliced
4 oz. pecans
4 oz. raisins
2 oz. sesame seeds

On a serving dish place the apple slices. Place a few pecans on top of the apple. Then sprinkle some raisins and sesame seeds on top. Serve.

VEGETABLE COCKTAIL

2 medium size carrots
1 celery stick
1 small cucumber
  Clump of watercress

Juice everything together and serve.

FRESH VEGETABLE JUICE

1 celery stick
2 medium size carrots
1 large tomato, cut in half

1 sweet red pepper, cut in half (stem, center, and seeds removed)
Small clump of red or green cabbage, cut in half

Juice everything together and serve.

GOURMET KASHA

4 oz. kasha, also known as buckwheat (preferably the whole granulation variety)
2 celery sticks, diced
1 small onion, diced
1 clove garlic, minced
1 cup water

Put water in a cooking pot and bring to a boil. Add ingredients and stir well. For a thinner texture add more water. For a thicker texture add more kasha. Cook until tender, then serve.

KIDNEY BEAN SUPREME

6 oz. kidney beans (soaked overnight)
3 oz. barley
3 celery sticks, diced
2 green bell peppers, diced (stem, center, and seeds removed)
1 small onion, diced
1 clove garlic, minced

Rinse barley and put in a cooking pot. Rinse kidney beans and then place beans in the same pot with the barley. Add fresh water. Add the celery, pepper, onion, and garlic and stir well. Cook for 30 to 40 minutes or until tender. Add more water if necessary. Serve.

NATURAL TOMATO SAUCE

2 medium size red ripe tomatoes, cut in half
½ green bell pepper, chopped finely (stem, center, and seeds removed)
2 oz. onion, chopped finely
½ clove garlic, minced
Pinch of thyme
Pinch of oregano

Put all the ingredients in a food processor or blender and blend well. Then pour contents in a cooking pot and cook for 20 to 30 minutes or until a desired texture is reached. Serve.

LUSCIOUS FRUIT SALAD

1 red delicious apple (or other sweet tasting apple), sliced
1 large sweet pear, sliced
2 large ripe peaches, sliced
2 large ripe plums, sliced
1 large ripe nectarine, sliced
½ pound green grapes

Place grapes in center of plate. Around the grapes, place the slices of fruit.

FROZEN BANANA-DATE PIE

3 bananas, sliced
1 pound pitted dates

Slice bananas and spread them on a pie dish. The sliced bananas will take the place of a pie crust. Then place dates in a food processor or blender. Add a little warm water and blend for a few minutes. Then pour contents on top of bananas and put in freezer. Keep in freezer for 2 hours. Serve.

POTATO SALAD

3 potatoes, lightly steamed
3 celery sticks, diced
3 cucumbers, diced
2 scallions, diced
2 green bell peppers, diced (stem, center, and seeds removed)
½ clove garlic, minced (optional)
    Fresh parsley or parsley flakes

Wash and steam potatoes until tender. After potatoes cool, peel and discard the skins. Cut the potatoes into small pieces and place in a bowl. Then add the other ingredients. Mix. Serve.

MIXED BEANS

2 oz. large lima beans (soaked overnight)
2 oz. pinto beans (soaked overnight)
2 oz. navy beans (soaked overnight)
2 oz. kidney beans (soaked overnight)
1 celery stick, diced
1 green bell pepper, diced (stem, center, and seeds removed)
1 small onion, diced
1 clove garlic, minced

Rinse beans and put in a cooking pot. Add fresh water. Add the celery, pepper, onion, and garlic and stir well. Cook for 30 to 40 minutes or until tender. Add more water if necessary. Serve.

TANGY COMPOTE

4 oz. dried apricots
4 oz. pitted prunes
4 oz. raisins
2 cups water

Place apricots, prunes, and raisins in a jar or a bowl. Pour in 2 cups of water. Let soak for 8 hours. When ready to eat, pour contents in a dessert dish and serve. (Note: Do not drain the water, the water which became a syrup is served as part of the dessert.) A delicious treat!

CHUNKY POTATO SOUP

4 small potatoes, peeled, then diced
4 oz. barley
1 celery stick, diced
1 green bell pepper, diced (stem, center, and seeds removed)
2 oz. zucchini, diced
2 oz. string beans, diced
2 oz. sweet green peas
1 small onion, diced
2 cloves garlic, minced
   Fresh parsley or parsley flakes

Put everything in a large cooking pot. Add water, stir, and cook for 40 minutes or until tender. Add more water if necessary. Serve. For extra taste, add parsley.

NOTES

CHAPTER 4.
A 6-WEEK EATING PLAN
FOR A TOXIC-FREE BODY

1. Herbert M. Shelton, *The Hygienic System, Vol. II* (San Antonio: Dr. Shelton's Health School, 1956), pp. 475-476.

2. *The Hygienic System, Vol. II*, p. 474.

3. *The Hygienic System, Vol. II*, p. 427.

4. Kurt J. Isselbacher, et al., *Harrison's Principles of Internal Medicine, Ninth Edition* (New York: McGraw-Hill, 1980), p. 433.
   Earl Mindell, *Vitamin Bible* (New York: Warner, 1985), p. 88.

5. Stephen Davies and Alan Stewart, *Nutritional Medicine* (New York: Avon Books, 1990), pp. 94, 385.
   Ronald L. Hoffman, *7 Weeks to a Settled Stomach* (New York: Pocket Books, 1991), p. 67.

5

A QUICKER WAY TO ACHIEVE A TOXIC-FREE BODY

Although the eating of fruits, especially oranges, grapefruit, tomatoes, grapes, and apples are the best foods that rid the body of toxins, Shelton claimed that "fasting," eating no food, is the quickest method of eliminating toxins from the body. In his childhood, Shelton observed that animals do not eat when they are sick. He said that when animals recover, their appetites return and they start eating again. Shelton referred to fasting as "nature's cure." He concluded that since animals benefit from fasting, humans can also benefit.[1]

The term fasting, as discussed here, means to voluntarily abstain from food, except pure water-preferably distilled water. Water enables the body to do many things that food cannot do. Overall, fasting provides the body with excellent conditions under which it can improve and restore health. According to Dr. Philip C. Royal, a fasting specialist who supervises fasts at the Hygiea-West Health Spa, fasting is a comfortable experience for most people. Dr. Royal says, "There is no easier way to make the transition to a more healthful lifestyle than by fasting."[2]

Without getting too technical, here is what goes on in the body during a fast: The fast provides a physiological rest for the body, permitting it to facilitate healing. The processes of digestion and assimilation of food are suspended, allowing the body to eliminate toxins at an increased rate. If disease has not reached an irreversible state, old and unhealthy cells are renewed and regenerated.

During the fast, the body consumes its nutritional reserves of fat, connective tissue, and muscle. The reduction of these tissues especially fat and connective tissue results in the liberation of stored toxins. These toxins are released into the bloodstream where they are then filtered out and removed from the blood. The process of fasting also lowers blood pressure.[3]

After several days of fasting, there is little or no desire for food.[4] The body consumes as fuel, excess fat and abnormal deposits.[5] According to Dr. Royal, "Weight loss in one week may be as much as 10 pounds or more."[6] Dr. Royal also found that most people who fasted reported an increase in mental acuity.[7] To sum it up in Dr. Shelton's words, "Fasting is the best, shortest, sharpest and fastest way to rid the body of toxins."[8]

A Three-Week Menu (With Fasting)

This is a three week regimen. In the first week, you fast for three continuous days (only drinking pure water, preferably distilled water). The menu I present shows the three consecutive fast days occurring on Tuesday, Wednesday, and Thursday in the first week of the three-week menu.

It is not essential that the fasting be done during the first week. This menu is flexible in the sense that you may schedule your own fasting program. If you wish, you may fast three consecutive days in the second or third week. The important thing to remember is to fast three consecutive days during this three-week period.

If you have any medical conditions or if you are taking any medications check with your physician before embarking on this fasting program. It is not advisable to fast for more than three consecutive days without professional supervision. If you want to detoxify under professional supervision consult with a Natural Hygiene practitioner, or stay at a detoxification spa (see Appendix 3 for a list of Natural Hygiene practitioners and detoxification spas).

This three-week menu, like the six-week menu, is not rigid with regards to quantities. You do not have to restrict portions; you may eat until you are satisfied (except of course, on fast days, where only water is permitted). And like the eating guidelines given for the six-week menu, when certain foods are not available, you may replace them with similar foods. However, be sure that you are not replacing the important fruits (oranges, grapefruit, tomatoes, grapes, and apples) that are necessary to rid the body of toxins. Before following the three-week menu please review the general guidelines given for the six-week menu in the previous chapter.

Preparations for foods denoted with asterisks (*)
are described at the end of Chapter 4.

1st Week

Sunday

BREAKFAST	LUNCH	DINNER
Grapefruit	*Fresh Vegetable Juice*	*Scrumptious Vegetable Salad*
Oranges	*Tasty Pita Sandwich*	*Great Tasting Baked Potatoes*
	Healthy Dressing	Steamed Cauliflower

Monday

BREAKFAST	LUNCH	DINNER
Apples	*Tropical Fruit Juice*	*Crispy Green Salad*
Peaches	*Luscious Fruit Salad*	*Healthy Dressing*
Bananas	Sunflower Seeds	*Tempting Strawberry Dessert*
	Pumpkin Seeds	Almonds

Tuesday: FAST

(no food, just distilled water)

Wednesday: FAST

(no food, just distilled water)

Thursday: FAST

(no food, just distilled water)

Friday

BREAKFAST

Orange Juice
and/or
Grapefruit Juice

LUNCH

Tropical Fruit Juice
Luscious Fruit Salad

DINNER

Scrumptious Vegetable Salad
Healthy Dressing
Apple Nut A La Mode

Saturday

BREAKFAST

Cantaloupe

LUNCH

Delectable Avocado Sandwich
Luscious Fruit Salad
Pistachio Nuts

DINNER

Scrumptious Vegetable Salad
Almonds
Filberts

2nd Week

Sunday

BREAKFAST

Apples
Nectarines
Plums

LUNCH

Crispy Green Salad
Easy Rice
Guilt-Free Blueberry Pie

DINNER

Exquisite Vegetable Stew
Baked Yams
Steamed String Beans

Monday

BREAKFAST

Grapes
Cherries
Kiwi fruit

LUNCH

Vegetable Cocktail
Zesty Peanut Butter Sandwich
Fantastic Split Pea Soup

DINNER

Scrumptious Vegetable Salad
Healthy Dressing
Whole Wheat Spaghetti
Natural Tomato Sauce

Tuesday

BREAKFAST	LUNCH	DINNER
Fresh Pineapple	*Crispy Green Salad*	*Scrumptious Vegetable Salad*
	Gourmet Kasha	*Great Tasting Baked Potatoes*
	Steamed Asparagus	Steamed Artichokes

Wednesday

BREAKFAST	LUNCH	DINNER
Papayas	*Tasty Pita Sandwich*	*Scrumptious Vegetable Salad*
Apricots	*Healthy Dressing*	*Barley Mushroom Soup*
Peaches	*Chickpea Savory*	*Tempting Strawberry Dessert*

Thursday

BREAKFAST	LUNCH	DINNER
Oranges	*Fresh Vegetable Juice*	*Scrumptious Vegetable Salad*
Grapefruit	*Luscious Fruit Salad*	*Healthy Dressing*
	Pistachio Nuts	*Mixed Beans*
		Steamed Cauliflower

Friday

BREAKFAST	LUNCH	DINNER
Mangos	*Chunky Potato Soup*	*Crispy Green Salad*
Peaches	Steamed Okra	*Apple Nut A La Mode*
	Steamed Zucchini	Filberts
	Steamed Sweet Green Peas	

Saturday

BREAKFAST	LUNCH	DINNER
Watermelon	*Delectable Avocado Sandwich*	*Scrumptious Vegetable Salad*
	Sunflower Seeds	Whole Grain Bread
	Almonds	Apples

3rd Week

Sunday

BREAKFAST   LUNCH   DINNER

*Tropical   *Crispy Green Salad*   *Kidney Bean Supreme*
 Fruit Juice* *Luscious Fruit Salad*   Steamed Broccoli
              Tangy Compote   Steamed String Beans

Monday

BREAKFAST   LUNCH   DINNER

Cantaloupe   *Vegetable Ambrosia*   *Scrumptious Vegetable Salad*
Honeydew   *Tasty Pita Sandwich*   *Delicious Corn*
              Healthy Dressing   Whole Grain Bread
              Apples   With Peanut Butter

Tuesday

BREAKFAST   LUNCH   DINNER

Persimmons   *Scrumptious Vegetable Salad*   *Barley Mushroom Soup*
Grapes   *Healthy Dressing*   Steamed Squash
Apples   Whole Wheat Macaroni   Steamed Okra
              Natural Tomato Sauce   Baked Sweet Potatoes

Wednesday

BREAKFAST   LUNCH   DINNER

Orange Juice *Fresh Vegetable Juice* *Scrumptious Vegetable Salad*
and/or   *Luscious Fruit Salad*   *Gourmet Kasha*
Grapefruit Juice *Frozen Banana-Date Pie* Steamed Cauliflower

Thursday

BREAKFAST	LUNCH	DINNER
Blueberries	*Delectable Avocado Sandwich*	*Scrumptious Vegetable Salad*
Strawberries	*Potato Salad*	*Healthy Dressing*
Tangerines	Steamed Sweet Green Peas	*Hearty Lentil Stew*

Friday

BREAKFAST	LUNCH	DINNER
Apples	*Crispy Green Salad*	*Scrumptious Vegetable Salad*
Pears	*Adzuki Rice Delight*	Almonds
Grapes	Sliced Apples Sprinkled	Sunflower Seeds
	With Hulled Sesame Seeds	

Saturday

BREAKFAST	LUNCH	DINNER
Oranges	*Scrumptious Vegetable Salad*	*Luscious Fruit Salad*
Grapefruit	*Zesty Peanut Butter Sandwich*	*Tasty Pita Sandwich*
Tangerines	Peaches	*Apple Nut A La Mode*

NOTES

CHAPTER 5.
A QUICKER WAY
TO ACHIEVE A TOXIC-FREE BODY

1. Jean A. Oswald, *Yours For Health: The Life and Times of Herbert M. Shelton* (Franklin, Wisconsin: Franklin Books, 1989), p. 12.

2. Dr. Philip C. Royal's Literature on Hygiea-West Health Spa.

3. *Yours For Health*, p. 82.

4. Dr. Philip C. Royal's Literature on Hygiea-West Health Spa.

5. *Yours For Health*, p. 82.

6-7. Dr. Philip C. Royal's Literature on Hygiea-West Health Spa.

8. *Yours For Health*, p. 58.

6

THE TOXIC-FREE COOKBOOK

After following the 6-week menu or 3-week menu, you may include these recipes in your diet. These recipes are wholesome and delicious!

The following recipes are furnished with permission by **Susan Taylor and** *Health Science* **magazine, the official membership journal of the American Natural Hygiene Society, Tampa, Florida.**

PEERLESS POTATO SALAD

    4 potatoes, lightly steamed
    1 small head of broccoli, steamed or raw
    4 stalks celery, diced
    2 avocados, mashed
      Romaine lettuce leaves

Wash and steam potatoes until tender. Cut into small pieces after cooling. Cut broccoli into small pieces, or divide flowerettes into individual pieces. Mix broccoli and diced celery with cut potatoes.

Cut avocados in half and remove flesh. Mash in small bowl and add to potato mixture. Toss until ingredients are tastefully mixed.

Use individual lettuce leaves to hold servings or tear lettuce into small pieces and add to salad.

STUFFED RED PEPPERS WITH AVOCADO STUFFING

1 sweet red pepper per guest, plus a few extra
1 avocado per pepper if avocado is small, or
½ avocado per pepper if avocado is large
   Sweet red peppers, diced
   Broccoli, finely chopped
   Celery, minced
   (Amounts of additional red peppers, broccoli and celery should be relative to number of peppers you are preparing)
   Cucumbers and carrots for garnish

Wash and remove tops and seeds from sweet peppers. Mash avocados and mix with diced peppers, broccoli and celery. Stuff each whole pepper with mixture.

Note: This procedure can be adapted for stuffing tomatoes as well. Add what you scooped out of the tomato to avocado mixture.

Serve on individual plates lined with lettuce leaves. Place stuffed pepper or tomato in center.

AVOCADO DRESSING

1 large or
2 small avocados
1 tomato

Cut avocado(s) in half, remove seed and scoop out the flesh. Be careful not to scoop too close to the skin, and remove any spotted or discolored avocado. Place in blender.

Cut tomato into wedges and add to the avocado in the blender. Blend at a low speed until mixture is smooth.

AVOCADO CELERY DRESSING

1 large or 2 small avocados
⅓ cup celery juice
1 teaspoon lemon or lime juice

Cut avocado(s) in half, remove seed and scoop out the flesh. Place in blender. Add freshly squeezed lemon or lime juice and celery juice, and blend everything together at a low speed until smooth and creamy. For a thick consistency add more avocado, for a thin consistency add more celery juice. If you want a strong flavor, add another teaspoon of lemon or lime juice.

CUCUMBER AVOCADO DRESSING

2 large cucumbers
1 large or 2 small avocados

Slice cucumbers into small pieces and mix in blender until smooth. Cut avocado(s) in half and remove pit. Scoop out the flesh and add to blended cucumbers. Blend entire mixture until smooth.

CRUNCHY AVOCADO DRESSING

2 large avocados
2 stalks celery
1 red pepper
Distilled water (add if you use a blender for the avocados)

Slice the avocados in half and remove the pits. Gently scoop out the flesh, avoiding the skin. Mash with a fork until smooth or blend in blender with just enough distilled water to get the sauce going. If you mash the avocado, it is not necessary to add distilled water.

Dice the celery and red pepper and mix in with the mashed or blended avocado. Simple and delicious!

The following recipes are furnished by **Dr. Keki R. Sidwa, President of the British Natural Hygiene Society and Director of the Shalimar Retreat, Essex, England.**

SHALIMAR SAVOURY

1 lb. very ripe small tomatoes
1 onion, finely chopped
1 small green or red pepper, finely chopped
1½ cups of grated carrots
1 cup soya flour
8 oz. tofu
1 tablespoon dried mixed herbs
1 tablespoon vegebase

Cook the tomatoes, carrots, onion, and pepper in a small amount of water. Then add soya flour, herbs and vegebase and cook for about 5 minutes. Put into a baking dish and add tofu on top. Bake in oven for 20 minutes at a moderate temperature. Dish can be served hot or cold.

MANGO ICE CREAM

2 large ripe mangos
½ lb. ground cashew nuts
½ pint apple juice

Peel the skins and remove pulp from the mangos. Discard the mango pits. Put mango pulp into food processor or blender and add the cashews and apple juice. After blending, pour contents onto a tray and then place tray in freezer. Keep in freezer until frozen. Remove tray from freezer ½ hour before eating. Mango ice cream is a delicious treat for young and old.

The following recipes are furnished by **Dr. Philip Martin, Toronto, Canada**.

TOMATO VEGETABLE SOUP

2 lbs. fresh or frozen vegetable assortment-cauliflower, broccoli, zucchini, peas, beans, and carrots. The 2 lbs. of vegetables should consist of equal portions.
1 quart fresh tomato juice

Combine all the ingredients. Put in cooking dish and bring to a boil. In the above recipe you may delete some vegetables to suit your taste or to achieve desired food combining.

BAKED EGGPLANT DELIGHT

1 eggplant
2 stalks celery, chopped
¼ red pepper, chopped
¼ green pepper, chopped
¼ yellow pepper, chopped

Pierce eggplant with knife. Then bake eggplant at 400 degrees for 1 hour. Peel and mash. When cool, add the celery and peppers. Serve with lettuce and sliced tomatoes.

The following recipe is furnished by **Jo Willard, President of Natural Hygiene, Inc., Shelton, Connecticut.**

PINEAPPLE AMBROSIA

(Serves 4)

> 1 ripe pineapple
> ½ cup sesame seeds
> 1 cup sunflower seeds (quantities of seeds may vary to suit your taste)

> Prepare and blend pineapple in blender or food processor. Remove from blender and pour into large bowl. Add sunflower seeds and sesame seeds and mix well. Place in small glass jars. Soak overnight. The dormant seeds start to activate due to the bromelain enzyme in the pineapple, making the food more easily digestible. Chew slowly, thoroughly and lovingly. Use for breakfast, lunch or supper.

The following recipes are furnished by **Dr. Douglas N. Graham, Director of Club Hygiene, Marathon, Florida.**

GREEK SALAD

(Serves 1)

> 2 tomatoes, diced
> 1 zucchini, diced
> 1 cup sprouts
> 1 red bell pepper, finely chopped
> ½ cup okra, chopped
> 12 ripe black olives (unsalted)
> ½ cup water

In a salad bowl, mix together tomatoes, zucchini, sprouts, pepper and okra. Blend olives with water in a blender or food processor to make a dressing. Pour dressing over salad and toss.

BROCCOMOLE SALAD

(Serves 2)

> 1½ cups red bell pepper, finely chopped
> 3 cups broccoli, finely chopped
> 1½ cups leaf lettuce, chopped
> 1 avocado, peeled and seed removed
> Lime juice to taste

In a salad bowl, mix together pepper, broccoli and lettuce. Blend avocado and lime juice in a blender or food processor, then pour over salad.

RAINBOW SALAD

(Serves 2)

> 1½ cups grated beets
> 1½ cups grated carrots
> 1½ cups grated yellow squash
> 1½ cups grated broccoli
> 1½ cups grated red cabbage

Arrange grated vegetables in rainbow-arched rows on a large platter. Serve with your choice of dressing.

SWEET RUSSIAN DRESSING

> 3 ripe tomatoes
> 1 large red bell pepper
> 1 avocado

Squeeze of lime juice

Place all the ingredients in a blender or food processor and blend.

TOMATO-WALNUT DRESSING

3 tomatoes
Raw walnuts (shells removed)

Blend until desired consistency is reached.

CASHEW-CUCUMBER DRESSING

2 cucumbers (peel removed)
Raw cashew pieces

Soak raw cashew pieces in water for several hours. Then drain the cashews. Put the cashews in a blender and then add the cucumbers. Blend until a desired consistency is reached.

HAWAIIAN CRUSH

(Serves 2)
6 oranges
1 fresh pineapple, peeled, cored and sliced
¼ cup raw nuts
Distilled water (optional)

Juice oranges and put juice in a blender with pineapple. Add nuts and blend until frothy. If too thick, add distilled water.

CREAMY FRUIT SHAKE

(Serves 2 or 3)

3 bananas, peeled, cut into chunks and frozen
3 fresh bananas, peeled
1 papaya, peeled and sliced
2 cups distilled water

Combine all the ingredients in a blender. Blend until smooth.

The following recipes are furnished by **Rhoda Mozorosky, Director of the Umpqua House, Roseburg, Oregon.**

BEET SOUP

1 peeled beet, diced
1 cup distilled water
½ avocado
½ lemon (squeezed)

Blend beet and water in blender, add avocado and lemon juice. Blend well and serve immediately in small soup bowls.

CUCUMBER SOUP

1 peeled cucumber, cut into large pieces
¼ cup distilled water
½ avocado
½ lemon (squeezed)
Scallions

Place all ingredients, except scallions in food processor or blender and blend well. Pour contents in small bowls. Then as a decoration, add finely chopped scallions on top of soup.

HEALTH GRANOLA

3 cups roll oats
1 cup pumpkin seeds
1 cup ground sesame seeds
1 cup sunflower seeds
¼ cup almond oil
¼ cup fruit concentrate (juice)
1 cup chopped nuts
1 cup raisins

Mix together and place on cookie sheet. Then place in oven set at 200 degrees for 30 minutes to 1 hour or until lightly toasted.

SUNSHINE SALAD

Grated beets
Grated carrots
Grated red and green cabbage
Sprouts
Avocado, sliced
Tomatoes, sliced

Place mound of beets in center of plate, circle with green cabbage, carrots, and red cabbage. Place sprouts around the plate. Decorate the sprouts with sliced tomatoes and sliced avocados.

The following recipes are furnished by **Bernice and Shirley Davison, Directors of the Health Oasis, Tilly, Arkansas.**

TOMATO FRENCH DRESSING

½ cup olive oil
⅓ cup lemon juice, freshly squeezed
¾ cup thick tomato juice

Shake well in tightly closed bottle and serve. You may include your favorite herb seasoning if you prefer more flavors.

PITA BREAD

2 packages dry yeast
1 ½ cups warm water
3 ½ to 4 cups whole wheat flour

In a large bowl, blend yeast and water. Let sit 5 minutes or until yeast is dissolved. Stir in 2 cups of flour. Gradually stir in remaining flour until a stiff dough forms.

On a lightly floured board, knead until smooth and elastic. Then place the dough in an oiled bowl, cover and let rise until doubled (1 to 2 hours). Punch dough down and turn on lightly floured board. Divide in 12 parts. Roll each ball into a thin circle, about 5 inches in diameter. Place the flattened rounds on a baking sheet. Let rise 20 to 30 minutes. Rounds will become fluffy. Bake until browned. Cool on rack. Freezes well. To reheat put in 350 degree oven until warm.

LENTILS WITH WALNUTS

(Serves 3)
2 cups lentils, uncooked
4 cups water
2 tablespoons oil
¼ teaspoon thyme
¾ cup walnuts, chopped

Use 4 cups of water to cook lentils until tender and quite dry. Put through a colander or mash. Add the walnuts and thyme. Then place in an oiled casserole dish and let it bake 20 to 30 minutes at 350 degrees.

CARROT SALAD

3 cups shredded carrots
½ cup chopped pecans
½ cup unsweetened pineapple chunks or crushed
½ cup chopped dates or raisins
3 tablespoons orange juice concentrate

Mix all the ingredients together and chill before serving.

GARDEN SLAW

1 cup shredded rutabaga
1 cup shredded cabbage
1 cup shredded carrots
  Chopped onion to taste
  Watercress

Toss vegetables together lightly and serve.

CUCUMBER SALAD

2 cucumbers, diced
3 or 4 celery stalks, chopped
1 quart fresh alfalfa sprouts, chopped
4 avocados, diced
  Juice of 1 lemon, for added taste

Toss and enjoy.

GREEN SALAD BOWL

1 head lettuce, chopped (or similar amount of other salad greens such
  as chicory, endive, escarole, romaine, raw spinach or watercress)

1 cucumber, thinly sliced
2 stalks celery, thinly diced
6 radishes, thinly sliced
3 tomatoes, cut up

Toss gently in large bowl and serve with any of the salad dressings listed in this book.

RICE VEGETABLE SALAD

3 cups brown rice, cooked and cold
1 cup peas and carrots, diced and steamed
½ cup celery, chopped
4 tablespoons cucumbers, diced

Toss and serve.

RED TOMATO SALAD

1 large tomato, cut in a flowerette
1 ripe avocado, mashed
Clump of alfalfa sprouts

Gently open the tomato. Place a scoop of mashed avocado in the center and top with alfalfa sprouts. For added taste, sprinkle with a few drops of lemon.

EASY PEA SOUP

1 pound green split peas
2 medium size onions
3 pints water
2 garlic cloves, minced (optional)

Combine all the ingredients and cook peas until tender (about 45 minutes). Serve with the salad of your choice.

7

NONTOXIC SOURCES OF VITAMINS

This chapter provides a list of the best sources for vitamins and minerals. You will find that vitamins and minerals are often found in abundance in raw fruits and vegetables, whole grains, nuts, seeds, and legumes. Although there are foods which contain high concentrations of vitamins and minerals, it is important to obtain vitamins and minerals in terms of quality instead of quantity.

Even though three ounces of beef liver contain more than five times the amount of vitamin A than three ounces of carrots, it is more healthful to obtain vitamin A by eating carrots. Unlike beef liver, carrots do not contain saturated fat or cholesterol. Here is another case in point: Three ounces of swiss cheese contain more than seven times the amount of calcium than three ounces of tofu. It is, however, more healthful to obtain your calcium requirements by eating tofu. Unlike swiss cheese, tofu does not contain saturated fat or cholesterol.

Anti-oxidant vitamins-A, C, and E, and the mineral selenium are crucial for maintaining a toxic-free body. Vitamins A, C, E, and the mineral selenium help prevent free radicals from forming in the body. Free radicals are highly reactive substances that cause damage to cells and tissues in the body. Without adequate supplies of vitamins A, C, E, and the mineral selenium, the body is susceptible to the damaging effects of free radicals. Cumulative damage to the cells and tissues cause illnesses and diseases.

In addition to vitamins A, C, E, and the mineral selenium, other vitamins and minerals are necessary for the body to function at an optimum level. Vitamins and minerals work along with the anti-oxidants to help speed the detoxification process.

City dwellers, those working with metals, and others who are routinely exposed to toxic pollutants need an increased amount of vitamins, especially the anti-oxidants.

Vitamin C and the B vitamins are water soluble. That is, they are not stored in the body for any real length of time (they are stored in the body for a few hours). Vitamins A, D, E, and K are fat soluble. These vitamins are stored in the body for a long period (except for vitamin E, fat soluble vitamins are stored in the body for a few days). Though vitamin E is a fat soluble vitamin, it remains in the body for a short period, much like the water soluble vitamins.

Heat and oxidation destroy certain vitamins. Don't overcook foods rich in vitamin B1 (Thiamine), Pantothenic Acid (vitamin B5, also part of the B-complex vitamins), Folic Acid (part of the B-complex vitamins), vitamin C (Ascorbic Acid), and vitamin E. Avoid soaking vegetables for more than a few minutes. Water leaches the B vitamins and vitamin C.

Also, don't leave foods rich in these vitamins exposed or uncovered for long periods. These guidelines do not apply to foods rich in minerals. Minerals generally lose only a fraction of their potency when cooked or left exposed.

Vitamins	Healthful Sources	Important For Maintaining Healthy
A (Beta carotene)	Carrots, cantaloupe, sweet potatoes, spinach, kale, broccoli, squash, apricots, pumpkin, mustard greens, watermelon, endive, green leafy vegetables, asparagus, peas, green beans, yellow corn.	Bones, Skin, Eyes, Hair
B1 (Thiamine, B-complex)	Brewer's yeast, nuts, seeds, brown rice, peas, beans, whole wheat, oatmeal, bran, most vegetables.	Nervous system, Brain, Muscles, Heart
B2 (Riboflavin, B-complex)	Brewer's yeast, yellow and green leafy vegetables, broccoli, peas, green beans, oats.	Skin, Hair, Eyes
B3 (Niacin, B-complex)	Brewer's yeast, whole grains, whole wheat, wheat germ, nuts, esp. peanuts, beans, avocados, dates, figs, prunes, most fruits and vegetables.	Nervous system, Brain, Skin

Vitamins	Healthful Sources	Important For Maintaining Healthy
B5 (Pantothenic Acid, B-complex)	Brewer's yeast, whole grains, wheat germ, nuts, most fruits and vegetables.	Digestive system, Nervous system, Brain, Heart
B6 (Pyridoxine)	Brewer's yeast, whole grains, wheat bran, wheat germ, cantaloupe, cabbage, bananas, potatoes, beans, cauliflower, most fruits and vegetables.	Nervous system, Muscles, Skin, Gums, Teeth
B12 (Cobalamin)	Brewer's yeast.	Nervous system, Blood, Bones, Skin, Muscles
Biotin (B-complex)	Brewer's yeast, nuts, brown rice, whole grains, cauliflower, peas, fruits, vegetables.	Skin, Muscles, Nervous system, Bones, Circulatory system
Choline (B-complex)	Brewer's yeast, whole grains, wheat germ, green leafy vegetables.	Nervous system, Brain
Folic Acid (B-complex)	Brewer's yeast, nuts, whole grains, whole wheat, bran, beans, cantaloupe, carrots, apricots, pumpkin, avocados, green leafy vegetables, fresh fruits.	Blood, Brain, Bones, Skin
Inositol (B-complex)	Brewer's yeast, wheat germ, dried lima beans, cantaloupe, grapefruit, raisins, peanuts, cabbage.	Blood, Brain, Muscles, Skin, Hair
PABA (Para-Aminobenzoic-Acid, B-complex)	Brewer's yeast, rice, bran, wheat germ.	Skin, Hair
C (Ascorbic acid)	Rose hips, citrus fruits, tomatoes, pineapple, strawberries, cabbage, spinach, potatoes, green peppers, sweet potatoes, berries, cauliflower, cherries, papaya, Brussels sprouts, broccoli, turnip greens.	Blood, Gums, Teeth, Skin, Bones
D	Sunlight.	Bones, Muscles, Nervous system, Skin, Heart, Teeth

Vitamins	Healthful Sources	Important For Maintaining Healthy
E (Tocopherol)	Nuts (almonds, pecans, hazelnuts, peanuts), seeds, esp. sunflower seeds, whole grains, wheat germ, whole wheat, soybeans, green leafy vegetables, spinach, Brussels sprouts, broccoli, cabbage.	Muscles, Skin, Lungs, Heart, Nervous system, Blood, Bones
K (Menadione)	Alfalfa, kelp, leafy green vegetables.	Blood

Minerals	Healthful Sources	Important For Maintaining Healthy
Calcium (Ca)	Soybeans, peanuts, walnuts, sunflower seeds, sesame seeds, dried beans, green leafy vegetables, broccoli, dandelion greens, collards, tofu, kale.	Blood, Bones, Teeth, Heart, Nervous system
Chloride (Cl)	Kelp.	Digestive system
Chromium (Cr)	Brewer's yeast, whole grains.	Blood
Cobalt (Co)	Seaweed.	Blood
Copper (Cu)	Whole grains, whole wheat, nuts, esp. almonds, dried legumes, leafy green vegetables, dried beans, peas, prunes.	Blood, Bones, Skin, Nervous system
Iodine (I)	Seaweed, kelp, and plants grown near the ocean where iodine content of soil is high.	Thyroid gland, Nervous system, Teeth, Hair, Nails, Skin
Iron (Fe)	Brewer's yeast, dried peaches, dried lima beans, dried kidney beans, dried soybeans, dried apricots, prunes, nuts, esp. almonds, asparagus, oatmeal, broccoli, spinach, peas, sunflower seeds, raisins, endive, escarole, beet greens, green leafy vegetables, whole wheat, corn.	Blood, Skin, Bones

Minerals	Healthful Sources	Important For Maintaining Healthy
Magnesium (Mg)	Fresh green vegetables, wheat germ, nuts, esp. almonds, cashews, Brazil nuts, pecans, peanuts, walnuts, seeds, soybeans, tofu, buckwheat (kasha), corn, whole wheat, oatmeal, black-eyed peas, kidney beans, bananas, beet greens, potatoes, avocados, apples, figs, lemons, grapefruit.	Nervous system, Heart, Teeth
Manganese (Mn)	Whole grains, nuts, green leafy vegetables, peas, beets.	Nervous system, Muscles, Bones
Molybdenum (Mo)	Green leafy vegetables, whole grains, legumes.	Blood
Phosphorus (P)	Whole grains, nuts, seeds, legumes, vegetables.	Bones, Teeth, Gums
Potassium (K)	Bananas, prunes, raisins, apricots, peaches, citrus fruits, cantaloupe, tomatoes, watercress, green leafy vegetables, winter squash, sunflower seeds, potatoes, avocados.	Nervous system, Muscles, Blood
Selenium (Se)	Whole grains, wheat germ, broccoli, tomatoes, onions, vegetables.	Skin, Hair
Sodium (Na)	Seaweed, kelp, tomatoes, celery, carrots, artichokes, beets, dandelion greens, kale, mustard greens, spinach.	Nervous system, Muscles
Sulfur (S)	Dried beans, cabbage, peas, lentils, mushrooms, Brussels sprouts.	Skin, Hair
Zinc (Zn)	Brewer's yeast, whole grains, wheat germ, pumpkin seeds, sunflower seeds, Brazil nuts, cashews, peanuts, soybeans, oats, peas, chickpeas (garbanzos), lentils.	Prostate gland, Blood

Vitamin/Mineral Supplements

Ideally you should obtain your daily vitamin and mineral requirements from the foods you eat. Remember, healthful sources of vitamins and minerals are found in raw fruits and vegetables, whole grains, nuts, seeds, and legumes.

On the healthy diet presented in this book, you receive all the vitamins and minerals necessary for creating a toxic-free body. This healthy diet, with its emphasis on fresh fruits and vegetables, foods that are naturally rich in vitamins (especially the anti-oxidant vitamins) and minerals, normally requires no supplements (except for vitamin B12 for certain individuals). Those who do not eat animal products may need to add a source of vitamin B12 to their diet (more on that later).

Vitamin and mineral supplements are not replacements for food. As the name suggests, they are supplemented to your meals. Vitamin and mineral supplements perform best when taken after large meals. If you take all your supplements at the same time, take them after eating your largest meal.

Here are some helpful hints for taking vitamin supplements. Because vitamins C, E, and the B vitamins do not accumulate in the body, they may be taken more frequently. If vitamins A, D, and K are taken in large doses they can cause harmful side effects. Unlike vitamin C, and the B vitamins, which are water soluble, and vitamin E which acts like a water soluble vitamin, excessive amounts of A, D, and K are not readily excreted by the body.

The Recommended Daily Allowance (RDA) for vitamin A is 5,000 International Units (I.U.) for most adults. One medium-sized carrot provides about four days worth of beta carotene which the body converts to vitamin A. Many people take 25,000 to 50,000 I.U. or more in daily supplements. Over a period, a daily dosage of 25,000 I.U. or more can cause liver damage, exopthalmus (abnormal protrusion of the eyeball from the orbit), joint pain and damage to the bones, dryness and fissures of the lips, and hair loss.[1]

Women who are pregnant or planning to become pregnant should check with a physician before taking vitamin A supplements. (Even if you are not a pregnant woman it is a good idea to consult your physician before taking vitamin A supplements.) Large doses of vitamin A have caused malformations in fetal animals. And large amounts of vitamin A (more than 25,000 I.U. a day) is suspected of causing malformations in human fetuses. Vitamin A toxicity does not result from eating plant sources such as carrots, cantaloupe, sweet potatoes, etc.

The RDA for vitamin D for most adults is 400 I.U. Daily requirement for this vitamin can be met by eating foods containing vitamin D precursors (yeast and plant foods) and by exposing your skin to sunlight for a short period so that the precursors can be activated.[2] Large doses of vitamin D (a daily intake of more than 25,000 I.U.) can cause permanent damage to the kidneys, heart, and blood vessels. Vitamin D toxicity does not result from eating plant precursors and exposing yourself to sunlight.

An overdose of vitamin K from animal or synthetic sources (tablets) can cause anemia. Like vitamin A and vitamin D, a vitamin K toxicity does not result from natural food sources. Vitamin K is found naturally in alfalfa, kelp, and green leafy vegetables. If you obtain your vitamins from healthful sources (plants and sunlight) you will not develop vitamin toxicities.

Before purchasing bottles of supplements check the labels. Make sure the vitamin/mineral tablets, capsules, or powder do not contain any of these ingredients:

Aluminum compounds	Sulfates
Animal sterates	Sulfites
Artificial flavors	Preservatives-BHA, BHT
Artificial colors	Salt fillers (sodium)
Starches	Sugars-fructose, sucrose

Those who are allergic to certain foods such as yeast, wheat, corn, soy products, or milk, should make sure the supplement is free of such ingredients. Vegetarians might be interested in checking the label for the sources of vitamins and minerals. Some vitamins and minerals list animal derivatives. For example, vitamin E may contain gelatin, calcium may be made from oyster shell, and minerals may be processed from bone meal.

Vitamin B12

Vitamin B12 is important for maintaining a healthy nervous system and promoting good blood circulation. This vitamin is mostly found in animal foods. Those who do not eat animal foods may need to add a source of vitamin B12 to their diet.

Before getting too concerned over vitamin B12 needs, it should be pointed out that vitamin B12 deficiency is a very rare occurrence.[3] The body accumulates at least a three-to-eight-year supply of this vitamin, so intake can occur sporadically without the risk of developing a deficiency.[4]

Those who avoid animal products can get their vitamin B12 requirement from other sources. Brewer's yeast is an ideal source.[5] Fermented soy products like tempeh contain sizable amounts of vitamin B12.[6] Also, sea vegetables such as kombu and wakame are excellent sources.[7] Brewer's yeast, fermented soy products, and sea vegetables (also known as sea weed) are available at health food stores.

Brewer's Yeast

As mentioned above, brewer's yeast can be a very nutritious food supplement. Do not purchase brewer's yeast if it contains preservatives, artificial flavors and colors, and sugar. Especially beware of aluminum! Some brands of brewer's yeast contain aluminum and may even promote it as a beneficial mineral.

Aluminum is a very undesirable ingredient. Human requirement for aluminum is non-existent. The body never needs aluminum. In no way can the consumption of aluminum bring about health benefits. As a matter of fact, consumption of aluminum is downright dangerous. Aluminum is recognized as being neuro-toxic; it has been implicated in brain disorders such as Alzheimer's disease.[8]

NOTES

CHAPTER 7.
NONTOXIC SOURCES OF VITAMINS

1. Kurt J. Isselbacher, et al., *Harrison's Principles of Internal Medicine, Ninth Edition* (New York: McGraw-Hill, 1980), p. 432.

2. John A. and Mary A. McDougall, *The McDougall Plan* (Piscataway, New Jersey: New Century, 1983), p. 136.

3-4. *The McDougall Plan*, pp. 39-40.

5. Stephen Davies and Alan Stewart, *Nutritional Medicine* (New York: Avon Books, 1990), pp. 22-23.

6. Lisa Tracy, *The Gradual Vegetarian* (New York: Evans, 1985), p. 103.

7. *The McDougall Plan*, p. 40.

8. *Nutritional Medicine*, pp. 94, 364, 385.
Ronald L. Hoffman, *7 Weeks to a Settled Stomach* (New York: Pocket Books, 1991), p. 67.

Appendix 1

Organic Food Resources

The term "organic" is generally defined as foods which have been grown using ecologically sound methods of farming. Synthetic pesticides, synthetic fertilizers, and growth stimulants are not used. Several states have enacted organic labeling laws and others have established statewide certification programs.

In 1990, both Houses of Congress passed a comprehensive national organic definition and certification bill. This legislation, incorporated into the 1990 Farm Bill, places organic products in the mainstream of the food industry. This bill applies to all foods claiming to be organically produced; it covers everything ranging from fresh fruits and vegetables to meats and poultry.

With a national definition of the term organic, backed by a certification process and supported by a national organic standards board, organic food is becoming a much respected product in the marketplace. This high level of public confidence in the "organically produced" label will convince more and more growers to switch to organic methods of farming.

The following **Organic Food-Mail Order Suppliers** ship their products directly to individual consumers, and do not require a minimum order unless otherwise stated. Write or call for their complete listings.

ARIZONA

Arjoy Acres
HCR Box 1410
Payson, AZ 85541
(602) 474-1224

Garlic, beans, peas, and fresh vegetables. (Fresh vegetables are available in the summer and fall.)

ARKANSAS

Dharma Farma
Star Route, Box 140
Osage, AR 72638
(501) 553-2550

Apples and pears.

Eagle Agricultural Products   Fresh and dried produce, beans, grains, pasta, cereals
407 Church Ave.   and flours.
Huntsville, AR 72740
(501) 738-2203

Good Earth Association   Corn, beans, and seeds.
202 E. Church St.
Pocahontas, AR 72455
(501) 892-9545
(501) 892-8329

Mountain Ark Trading Co.   Grains, beans, nuts, seeds, pasta, cereals, flours, sea
120 South East Ave.   vegetables (sea weed), and wide selection of Macrobi-
Fayetteville, AR 72701   otic items.
(800) 643-8909
(501) 442-7191

CALIFORNIA

Ahler's Organic Date Garden   Dates and date products.
P.O. Box 726
Mecca, CA 92254
(619) 396-2337

Blue Heron Farm   Almonds, walnuts, and oranges. Min. 5 lbs. almonds
P.O. Box 68   or walnuts; Min. 35 lbs. oranges. (Walnuts are avail-
Rumsey, CA 95679   able by late October; oranges are available by mid
(916) 796-3799   January. Write or call after January 1st for prices and
                                  shipping information on oranges.)

Buhler Pistachio Farms   Pistachio nuts. Specify organic. Min. 5 lbs.
1265 S. Lyon Ave.
Mendota, CA 93640
(209) 655-4949

Colvalda Date Co.   Dates, dried fruits, nuts, seeds, and citrus.
P.O. Box 908
Coachella, CA 92236
(619) 398-3441
FAX (619) 398-1615

Capay Fruits and Vegetables   Dried tomatoes, peaches, and herbs.
Star Route, Box 3
Capay, CA 95607
(916) 796-4111

Dach Ranch   Apples, apple products, and pears.
P.O. Box 44
Philo, CA 95466
(707) 895-3173

Ecology Sound Farms   Oranges, plums, Asian pears, kiwi fruit, and persim-
42126 Road 168   mons. Min. varies.
Orosi, CA 93647
(209) 528-3816
(209) 528-2276

Diamond Organics   Lettuce, greens, roots and tubers, squash, sprouts,
Freedom, CA 95019   herbs, mushrooms, citrus, apples, pears, and other
(800) 922-2396   fruits and vegetables.

Gold Mine Natural Food Co.   Grains, beans, cereals, flours, breads, seeds, soy
1947 30th St.   sauces, sea vegetables, teas, and large selection of
San Diego, CA 92102   Macrobiotic items.
In CA (800) 647-2927
Elsewhere in US (800) 647-2929
(619) 234-9711

G. Grell   Six varieties of avocados. Min. 25 lbs.
P.O. Box 7092
Halcyon, CA 93420
(805) 489-2227

Gravelly Ridge Farms   Produce and grains.
Star Route 16
Elk Creek, CA 95939
(916) 963-3216

Great Date in the Morning   Dates.
P.O. Box 31
Coachella, CA 92236
(619) 398-6171

Green Knoll Farm
P.O. Box 434
Gridley, CA 95948
(916) 846-3431

Kiwi fruit. Min. 7 ½ lbs.

Jaffe Bros.
P.O. Box 636
Valley Center, CA 92082
(619) 749-1133
FAX (619) 749-1282

Dried fruit, grains, cereals, flours, pasta, peas, beans, nuts, seeds, nut butters, jams, honey, juices, and other items. Min. varies.

Living Tree Centre
P.O. Box 10082
Berkeley, CA 94709
(415) 420-1440

Almonds, almond butter, and pistachio nuts. (Also sells apple, pear, and apricot trees.)

Lundberg Family Farms
P.O. Box 369
Richvale, CA 95974
(916) 882-4551

Rice and rice products.

Mendocino Sea Vegetable Co.
P.O. Box 372
Navarro, CA 95463
(707) 895-3741

Wildcrafted sea vegetables (seaweed).

Old Mill Farm School of
Country Living
P.O. Box 463
Mendocino, CA 95460
(707) 937-0244

Lamb, goat cheese, and produce. Min. $50.

Organic Food Shipper
352 Hilltop Dr.
Chula Vista, CA 92010
In CA (800) 225-8879
Elsewhere in US (800) 225-0852
(619) 425-2813

Fresh fruits and vegetables, dried fruit, seeds, grains, beans, nuts, and raw milk products.

Steven Pavich and Sons
Rt. 2, Box 291
Delano, CA 93215
(805) 725-1046

Grapes and melons.

Santa Cruz Orchards   Apples, apple juice, apple butter and apple sauce.
Box 1510
Freedom, CA 95019
(408) 728-0414

Sleepy Hollow Farm   Apples and herbs. Min. 40 lbs. for apples.
44001 Dunlap Rd.
Miramonte, CA 93641
(209) 336-2444

Joe Soghomonian   Grapes (available from August to September) and rai-
8624 S. Chestnut   sins (available year 'round). Min. 24 lbs. for grapes;
Fresno, CA 93725   Min. 6 lbs. for raisins.
(209) 834-2772
(209) 834-3150

Sun Gardens   Dates and date products. Specify organic.
P.O. Box 190
Bard, CA 92222
Outside California (800) 228-4690
Anywhere (including Calif.) (619) 572-0088

Timber Crest Farms   Dried tomatoes, dried fruit, fruit butters, and nuts.
4791 Dry Creek Rd.
Healdsburg, CA 95448
(707) 433-8251

Weiss's Kiwi Fruit   Kiwi fruit available from October to December. Min.
594 Paseo Companeros   2 ½ lbs.
Chico, CA 95928
(916) 343-2354

Your Land Our Land   Produce, herbs and garlic.
P.O. Box 485
Los Altos, CA 94022
(415) 821-6732

Van Dyke Ranch   Dried apricots and dried cherries. Min. 5 lbs.
7665 Crews Rd.
Gilroy, CA 95020
(408) 842-5423

Whelen Apple Farm   Apples and cider.
John S. Whelen
15300 Moro Rd.
Atascadero, CA 93422

The Worm Concern   Organically grown seeds, organic soil and fertilizer,
580 Erbes Rd.   worms and worm castings, and produce.
Thousand Oaks, CA 91362
(805) 496-2872

COLORADO

Malachite Small Farm School   Honey, quinoa, and beef.
ASR Box 21-Pass Creek Rd.
Gardner, CO 81040
(719) 746-2412

Wilton's Organic Potatoes   Potato seeds. Min. 5 lbs.
Box 28
Aspen, CO 81612
(303) 925-3433

CONNECTICUT

Butterbrooke Farm   75 varieties of vegetable seeds.
78 Barry Rd.
Oxford, CT 06483
(203) 888-2000

DISTRICT OF COLUMBIA

Tabard Farm Potato Chips   Potato chips.
1739 N St., NW
Washington, DC 20036
(202) 785-1277

FLORIDA

Sprout Delights
13090 NW 7th Ave.
Miami, FL 33168
(800) 334-2253
(305) 687-5880

Sprouted breads, rolls, muffins, brownies and cakes. Min. $20.

Starr Organic Produce, Inc.
P.O. Box 561502
Miami, FL 33256
(305) 262-1242

Large selection of fruits. Min. 20 lbs.

GEORGIA

Allos
P.O. Box 8450
Atlanta, GA 30306
(800) 648-6554

Exotic honey. Min. $15.

Michael's Mountain Honey
Michael Surles
Rt. 4, Box 826
Blairsville, GA 30512
(404) 745-4170

Honey and bee pollen.

Bricker's Organic Farm Inc.
824 Sandbar Ferry Rd.
Augusta, GA 30901
(404) 722-0661

Tomatoes and catfish.

HAWAII

Hawaiian Exotic Fruit Co.
Box 1729
Pahoa, HI 96778
(808) 965-7154

Dried pineapples, dried papayas, dried bananas, fresh ginger root, and turmeric. Min. 10 lbs.

IDAHO

Ronniger's Seed Potatoes   Potato seeds and potatoes. Min. 10 lbs. for potatoes.
Star Route
Moyie Springs, ID 83845
(208) 267-7938

Mountain Star Honey Co.   Honey, fruit mixtures, bee pollen, and maple syrup.
Kent and Sharon Wenkheimer
P.O. Box 179
Peck, ID 83545
(208) 486-6821

ILLINOIS

Green Earth Natural Foods   Fresh produce, meats, and large selection of other
2545 Prairie Ave.   items.
Evanston, IL 60201
(800) 322-3662
(312) 864-8949

Nu-World Amaranth   Amaranth flour, cereals, and whole grains.
P.O. Box 2202
Naperville, IL 60565
(312) 369-6819

Sunrise Farm Health Food Store Grains, nuts, seeds, dried fruit, juice, yeast, cheese,
17650 Torrence Ave.   vegetables, and other items.
Lansing, IL 60438
(312) 474-6166

INDIANA

Dutch Mill Cheese   Cheese. Min. 3 lbs.
2001 N. State Rd. I
Cambridge City, IN 47327
(317) 478-5847

IOWA

The Herb & Spice Collection
P.O. Box 118
Norway, IA 52318
(800) 365-4372

Herbs, spices, and teas.

Paul's Grains
2475-B 340 St.
Laurel, IA 50141
(515) 476-3373

Grains and grain products, flours, produce, honey, eggs, beef, lamb, chicken, and turkey.

Clarence Van Sant
Rt. 2
Grinell, IA 50112
(515) 526-8522

Grains, corn, soybeans, honey, eggs, and beef.

KENTUCKY

Gracious Living Farm
General Delivery
Insko, KY 41443

Vegetables.

LOUISIANA

Rein Farms
812 Cedar Ave.
Metairie, LA 70001
(504) 888-5763

Vegetables.

MAINE

Avena Botanicals
Deb Soule
P.O. Box 365
West Rockport, ME 04865
(207) 594-0694

Herbs. Retail catalog $1.50.

Crossroad Farms
Box 3230
Jonesport, ME 04649
(207) 497-2641

Root crops, squash, cabbage, strawberries, and 50 varieties of apples. Min. $25.

Fiddler's Green Farm
RFD 1, Box 656
Belfast, ME 04915
(207) 338-3568

Grains, cereals, flours, pasta, baking mixes, potatoes, jams, syrups, honey, coffee, teas, and organic baby foods.

Johnny's Selected Seeds
Foss Hill Rd.
Albion, ME 04910
(207) 437-9294

Vegetable seeds, herb seeds, and other seeds.

Maine Coast Sea Vegetables
Shore Rd.
Franklin, ME 04634
(207) 565-2907

Sea chips, kelp, dulse, and nori.

Ram Island Farm Herbs
Ram Island Farm
Cape Elizabeth, ME 04107
(207) 767-5700

Dried herbs.

Simply Pure Food
RFD 3, Box 99
Bangor, ME 04401
(800) IAM-PURE
(207) 941-1924

Strained and diced baby foods and baby cereals.

Wolfe's Neck Farm
RR 1, Box 71
Freeport, ME 04032
(800) 346-9540
(207) 865-4469

Beef. Min. 42 lbs.

WoodPrairie Farm
Jim and Megan Gerritsen
RFD 1, Box 164
Bridgewater, ME 04735
(207) 429-9765

Potatoes and vegetables.

MARYLAND

Macrobiotic Mall
18779-C N. Frederick Ave.
Gaithersburg, MD 20879
(800) 553-1270
(301) 963-9235

Grains, legumes, packaged foods, and large selection of Macrobiotic items.

Organic Foods Express
11003 Emack Rd.
Beltsville, MD 20705
(301) 937-8608

Produce, grains, beans, and large selection of other items.

Wilton's Organic Plants
Leroy J. Wilton
357 Catherine and Harlem Aves.
Pasadena, MD 21122
(301) 647-1488

Herbs, vegetable and flower plants. Catalog $2, deductible with order.

MASSACHUSETTS

Baldwin Hill Bakery
Baldwin Hill Rd.
Phillipston, MA 01331
(508) 249-4691

Sourdough bread. Min. 12 loaves.

Cooks Maple Products
Bashan Hill Rd.
Worthington, MA 01098
(413) 238-5827

Maple syrup.

The Sprout House
40 Railroad St.
Great Barrington, MA 01230
(413) 528-5200

A variety of seeds for sprouting.

White Oak Farm
c/o NE Small Farm Institute
Jepson House
Jackson St., Box 937
Belchertown, MA 01007
(413) 323-4531

Squash and dry beans.

MICHIGAN

American Spoon Foods
P.O. Box 566
Petoskey, MI 49770
In MI (800) 222-5886
Elsewhere in US (800) 327-7984
(616) 347-9030

Wild rice, wild pecans, hickory nuts, black walnuts, wild berry preserves, honey, and maple syrup.

Cosmic Realities
P.O. Box 1250
Jackson, MI 49204
(517) 783-2293

Sprouted foods, grains, and beans.

Country Life Natural Foods
109th Ave.
Pullman, MI 49450
(616) 236-5011

Beans, grains, seeds, nuts, and raisins.

Eden Foods
701 Tecumseh Rd.
Clinton, MI 49236
(517) 456-7424

A large variety of domestic and imported whole foods.

Eugene and Joan Saintz
2225 63rd St.
Fennville, MI 49408
(616) 561-2761

Fresh produce in season.

Richards Natural Food Farm
Richard and Janet Osterbeck
15213 Hinman Rd.
Eagle, MI 48822
(517) 627-7965

Eggs, turkey, vegetables, and elephant garlic.

Specialty Grain Co.
Box 2458
Dearborn, MI 48123
(313) 535-9222

Grains, beans, dried fruit, seeds, and nuts.

Sunshower
48548 60th Ave.
Lawrence, MI 49064
(616) 674-3103

Apples, pears, vegetables, fruit butters, juices, and lamb.

MINNESOTA

Diamond K. Enterprises
RR 1, Box 30A
St. Charles, MN 55972
(507) 932-4308
(507) 932-5433

Grains, flours, cereals, pancake mixes, nuts, sunflower seeds, alfalfa seeds, dried fruit, honey, and sunflower oil.

French Meadow Bakery
2610 Lyndale Ave., So.
Minneapolis, MN 55408
(612) 870-4740

Sourdough bread. Min. $20.

Living Farms
P.O. Box 50
Tracy, MN 56175
In MN (800) 622-5235
Elsewhere in US (800) 533-5320
(507) 629-4431

Grains, wheat, beans, sunflower seeds, and sprouting seeds (alfalfa, clover and radish).

Mill City Sourdough Bakery
1566 Randolph Ave.
St. Paul, MN 55105
(800) 87-DOUGH
(612) 698-4705

Sourdough bread. Min. 6 loaves.

Natural Way Mills, Inc.
Rt. 2, Box 37
Middle River, MN 56737
(218) 222-3677

Grains, flours, cereals, and other items.

MISSOURI

Morningland Dairy
Rt. 1, Box 188-B
Mountain View, MO 65548
(417) 469-3817

Raw milk cheeses.

NEBRASKA

Do-R-Dye Organic Mill   Oats, wheat, rye, and corn products. Min. $5.
Box 50
Rosalie, NE 68055
(402) 863-2248

M & M Distributing   Amaranth and blue corn products.
RR 2, Box 61A
Oshkosh, NE 69154
(308) 772-3664

Stapelman Meats   Beef.
Rt. 2, Box 6A
Belden, NE 68717
(402) 985-2470

NEW HAMPSHIRE

Apple Jacks Cider Mill   Apple cider and vinegar.
24 Francestown Rd.
New Boston, NH 03070

Water Wheel Sugar House   Maple syrup.
Rt. 2
Jefferson, NH 03583
(603) 586-4479

NEW JERSEY

Organically Yours   Fresh produce.
Paul Keiser and Nancy Jones
P.O. Box 186
Riverside, NJ 08075
(609) 786-2777

Simply Delicious   Large selection of items.
243 A N. Hook Rd., Box 124
Pennsville, NJ 08070
(609) 678-4488

NEW MEXICO

Estawanca Valley
Garlic Growers
P.O. Box 892
Moriarty, NM 87035
(505) 832-6177

Elephant garlic. Min. $10.

NEW YORK

Back of the Beyond
Shash Georgi and Bill Georgi
7233 Lower E. Hill Rd.
Colden, NY 14033
(716) 652-0427

Herb plants, herb honey and herb products. Limited shipping.

Bread Alone
Rt. 28
Boiceville, NY 12412
(914) 657-3328

Wheat, rye and sourdough bread. Min. 12 loaves.

Community Mill and Bean
RD 1, Rt. 89
Savannah, NY 13146
(315) 365-2664

Flours, cereals, grains, mixes, and beans. Min. $10.

Deer Valley Farm
RD 1
Guilford, NY 13780
(607) 764-8556

Beef, chicken, turkey, veal, lamb, eggs, produce, grains, pasta, soups, baked goods, nuts, oils, nut butters, jams, herbs and seasonings. Min. $10.

Four Chimneys Farm Winery
RD 1, Hall Rd.
Himrod, NY 14842
(607) 243-7502

Wine, grape juice, and wine vinegar. Min. 1 case of wine or grape juice.

NORTH CAROLINA

American Forest Foods Corp.
Rt. 5, Box 84E
Henderson, NC 27536
(919) 438-2674

Shiitake and oyster mushrooms, mixes, and spices. Min. 12 packs.

Briarpath Farm   Elephant garlic.
P.O. Box 548
Carrboro, NC 27510
(919) 998-3340

Natural Lifestyle Supplies   Grains, cereals, beans, pasta, nuts, seeds, nut butters,
16 Lookout Dr.   jams, sauces, dried fruit, sea vegetables, and wide se-
Asheville, NC 28804   lection of Macrobiotic items.
(800) 752-2775
(704) 254-9606

Patricia Pope   Honey.
Rt. 6, Box 76B
Mocksville, NC 27028

OHIO

Elias W. Keim   Vegetables, oats, and corn.
1488 T.R. 1008, Rt. 1
Ashland, OH 44805

Millstream Natural   Produce, nuts, grains, and cereals.
Health Supplies
1310A E. Tallmadge Ave.
Akron, OH 44310
(216) 630-2700

Sanctuary Farm   Grains, beans, and seeds. Min. 25 lbs.
RD 1, Butler Rd.
Box 184-A
New London, OH 44851
(419) 929-8177

OKLAHOMA

Earth Natural Foods and Deli   Grains, beans, nuts, fruits, apples, apple juice and
309 S. Flood   apple sauce, and herbs. Min. $25.
Norman, OK 73069
(405) 364-3551

OREGON

Dement Creek Farms
Box 155
Broadbent, OR 97414
(503) 572-5564

Beans, grains, vegetables, and herbs.

Herb Pharm
P.O. Box 116
Williams, OR 97544
(503) 846-7178

Herbs, herbal extracts, spices, and teas. Min. $25.

PENNSYLVANIA

Better Foods Foundation Inc.
200 N. Washington St.
Greencastle, PA 17265
(717) 597-7127

Selected items.

Bramble Hill Beefs
T.J. Moore
RD 1
Lucinda, PA 16235
(814) 354-2207

Beef.

Dutch Country Gardens
Joseph Yasenchak
RD 1, Box 1122
Tamaqua, PA 18252
(717) 668-0441

Potatoes and carrots. Min. $25.

Garden Spot Distributors
438 White Oak Rd.
New Holland, PA 17557
In PA (800) 292-9631
In Eastern US (800) 445-5100
(717) 354-4936

Cereals, grains, flours, beans, baked goods, dried
fruit, nuts, seeds, teas, and herbs.

Genesee Natural Foods
RD 2, Box 105
Genesee, PA 16923
(814) 228-3200
(814) 228-3205

Beans, grains, flours, cereals, pasta, seeds, dried fruit,
nut butters, pear and apple juice, and teas.

Krystal Wharf Farms
RD 2, Box 191A
Mansfield, PA 16933
(717) 549-8194

Grains, beans, nuts, dried fruit, fresh produce, and other items.

Rising Sun Distributors
P.O. Box 627
Milesburg, PA 16853
(814) 355-9850

Produce, meats, poultry, dairy products, grains, nuts, seeds, breads, beans, dried fruit, and other items.

Walnut Acres
Walnut Acres Rd.
Penns Creek, PA 17862
(800) 433-3998
FAX (717) 837-1146

Grains, cereals, flours, breads, beans, soups, pasta, nuts, seeds, dried fruit, sauces, jams and preserves, nut butters, salad dressings, fruits, vegetables, meats, dairy products, juices, herbs and spices.

RHODE ISLAND

Meadowbrook Herb Gardens
Wyoming, RI 02898
(401) 539-7603

Herbs and teas. Catalog $1.

TEXAS

Arrowhead Mills
Box 2059
Hereford, TX 79045
(806) 364-0730

Grains and grain products, beans, and seeds.

Carr's Specialty Foods
P.O. Box 1016
Manchaca, TX 78652
(512) 282-9056

Dried fruit, nuts, seeds, beans and peas, grains, flours, cereals and granolas, herbs and spices.

J. Francis Co.
Rt. 3, Box 54
Atlanta, TX 75551
(214) 796-5364

Pecans. Min. 5 lbs.

Hawkins Creek Farm
P.O. Box 6552
Longview, TX 75608
(214) 759-8820

Potatoes.

Stanley Jacobson
1505 Doherty
Mission, TX 78572
(512) 585-1712

Grapefruit and oranges. Min. 1/4 bushel.

Lee's Organic Foods
Box 111
Wellington, TX 79095
(806) 447-5445

Fruit jerkies and dried apples. Min. $5.

UTAH

Aquaculture Marketing Service
356 W. Redview Dr.
Monroe, UT 84754
(800) 634-5463, ext. 230
(801) 527-4528

Frozen, canned and smoked rainbow trout.

VERMONT

Gourmet Produce Co.
Richard Rommer
RR 3, Box 348
Chester, VT 05143
(802) 875-3820

Wheat grass, wheat grass juice, and sunflower sprouts.

Hill and Dale Farms
West Hill-Daniel Davis Rd.
Putney, VT 05346
(802) 387-5817

Apples, apple cider and apple vinegar. Min. 24 apples.

Teago Hill Farm
Barber Hill Rd.
Pomfret, VT 05067
(802) 457-3507

Maple syrup.

Tinmouth Channel Farm
Town Highway 19
Box 428 B
Tinmouth, VT 05773
(802) 446-2812

Herbs and herb plants. Catalog $1.

VIRGINIA

Blue Ridge Food Service
Rt. 3, Box 304
Edinburg, VA 22824
(703) 459-3379

Rainbow trout. Min. 5 lbs.

Golden Acres Orchard
Rt. 2, Box 2450
Front Royal, VA 22630
(703) 636-9611

Apples, apple cider, apple juice, and apple vinegar.

Golden Angels Apiary
P.O. Box 2
Singers Glen, VA 22850
(703) 833-5104

Five types of honey.

Kennedy's Natural Foods
1051 W. Broad St.
Falls Church, VA 22046
(703) 533-8484

Large selection of items.

Natural Beef Farms
4399-A Henninger Ct.
Chantilly, VA 22021
(703) 631-0881

Frozen meats, produce, breads, and large selection of other items.

WASHINGTON

Cascadian Farm
5375 Highway 20
Rockport, WA 98283
(206) 853-8175

Fruit preserves and dill pickles.

Homestead Organic Produce
Rt. 1, 2002 Rd. 7 NW
Quincy, WA 98848
(509) 787-2248

Sweet onions, Korean garlic, walnuts, filberts, red delicious and golden delicious apples, nuts, and dried fruit. Min. varies.

Sweet Wind Gardens
Richard Murray
Rt. 2, Box 540
Twisp, WA 98856
(509) 997-4891

Anise hyssop seed and garlic.

WEST VIRGINIA

Brier Run Farm   Goat cheeses.
Rt. 1, Box 73
Birch River, WV 26610
(304) 649-2975

Hardscrabble Enterprises, Inc.   Dried American shiitake mushrooms. Min. 1 ½ lbs.
Rt. 6, Box 42
Cherry Grove, WV 26804
(304) 567-2727
(202) 332-0232

WISCONSIN

Joel Afdahl   Maple syrup.
Rt. 1, Box 270
Hammond, WI 54015
(715) 796-5395

Nokomis Farm   Grains, flours, breads and bakery products, and beef.
3293 Main St.   Min. $50.
East Troy, WI 53120
(414) 642-9665

CANADA

A. Scheresky   Millet, oats, wheat, flours and other grains. Shipped
Box 240   anywhere in Canada and some points in US.
Oxbow, SK S0C 2B0
(306) 925-2114

Variety Acre Organic Gardening   Dried fruit, fruit leather, vegetables, herbs and season-
Howard and Netta Thompson   ings.
Box 117
Oliver, BC V0H 1T0
(604) 498-2445

Wholesale Organic Food Suppliers

The following is a list of wholesale organic food suppliers. These mail-order distributors require a large order. They sell a variety of items. You can save a lot of money on organic foods by buying in large quantities. It may be a good idea to get together with your friends and share an order. Write or call these distributors to find out what foods they sell, and what their minimum order is.

Appleseed Ranch/Sonoma Gold Organics
1834 High School Rd.
Sebastopol, CA 95472
(707) 829-1121

Bellevue Gardens Organic Farm
625 Bellevue Lane
Archer, FL 32618
(904) 495-2348

Blooming Prairie Natural Foods
510 Kasota Ave.
Minneapolis, MN 55414
(612) 378-9774

Blooming Prairie Warehouse
2340 Heinz Rd.
Iowa City, IA 52240
(319) 337-6448

Clear Eye Warehouse
RD 1, Rt. 89
Savannah, NY 13146
(315) 365-2816

Coke Farm
17245 Tarpey Rd.
Watsonville, CA 95076
(408) 726-3100

Common Health Warehouse
1505 N. 8th St.
Superior, WI 54880
(715) 392-9862

Federation of Ohio River Cooperatives
320 Outerbelt, Suite E
Columbus, OH 43213
(614) 861-2446

Genesee Natural Foods
RD 2, Box 105
Genesee, PA 16923
(814) 228-3200

Hudson Valley Federation
P.O. Box 367
Clintondale, NY 12515
(914) 883-6848

Michigan Federation of Food Cooperatives
727 W. Ellsworth #15
Ann Arbor, MI 48108
(313) 761-4642

Mountain Warehouse
1400 E. Geer St.
Warehouse #3
Durham, NC 27704
(919) 682-9234

Neshaminy Valley Natural Foods
5 Louise Dr.
Ivyland, PA 18974
(215) 443-5545

North Coast Cooperative
3134 Jacobs Ave.
Eureka, CA 95501
(707) 445-3185

Northeast Cooperatives
P.O. Box 1120
Quinn Rd.
Brattleboro, VT 05302
(802) 257-5856

North Farm Cooperative Warehouse
204 Regas Rd.
Madison, WI 53714
(608) 241-3995

Nutrasource
4005 6th Ave. S.
Seattle, WA 98108
(206) 467-7190

Orange Blossom Cooperative Warehouse
1601 NW 55th Pl.
Gainesville, FL 32609
(904) 372-7061

Organic Farms
10714 Hanna St.
Beltsville, MD 20705
In MD (800) 792-8344
Elsewhere in US (800) 222-6244
(301) 595-5151

Ozark Cooperative Warehouse
P.O. Box 30
Fayetteville, AR 72702
(501) 521-2667

Tucson Cooperative Warehouse
350 S. Toole
Tucson AZ 85701
(602) 884-9951

West Valley Produce Co.
726 S. Mateo St.
Los Angeles, CA 90021
(213) 627-4131

Organic Food Alliance

The Organic Food Alliance is a national organization that represents the Organic Food Industry in Washington, D.C. Its members include growers, manufacturers, distributors, retailers, consumers, and others who support organic farming. For more information about this organization and how to become a member contact:

Organic Food Alliance
2111 Wilson Blvd., Suite 531
Arlington, VA 22201
(703) 276-8009

Organic Associations

The following associations offer advice on organic farming methods. If you are interested in starting your own organic garden, these associations are eager to help you. They can provide you with information on disease resistance plants, beneficial insects, natural fertilizers, and other methods of organic farming. These associations will also try to answer any question you might have about organic gardening.

ARKANSAS

Ozark Organic Growers Association
Contact: Gordon Watkins
HCR 72, Box 34
Parthenon, AR 72666
(501) 446-5783

CALIFORNIA

California Certified Organic Growers
P.O. Box 8136
Santa Cruz, CA 95061
(408) 423-2263

Demeter Association
4214 National Ave.
Burbank, CA 91505
(818) 343-5521

CONNECTICUT

Farm Verified Organic
P.O. Box 45
Redding, CT 06875
(203) 544-9896

DISTRICT OF COLUMBIA

Universal Proutist Farmers Federation
1354 Montague, NW
Washington, DC 20011
(202) 882-8804

FLORIDA

Florida Organic Growers Association
Contact: Tim Logan
1920 SW 70th Terrace
Gainesville, FL 32607
(904) 332-3353

Alachua County Extension Office
Contact: Gary Brinen
2800 NE 39th Ave.
Gainesville, FL 32609

GEORGIA

Georgia Organic Growers Association
Contact: Diane Jerkins or Deborah
Pelham
P.O. Box 567661
Atlanta, GA 30356
Diane Jerkins (404) 378-7843
Deborah Pelham (404) 476-0473

ILLINOIS

IPM for the Home and Garden
Institute for Environmental Studies
University of Illinois
408 S. Goodwin Ave.
Urbana, IL 61801
(217) 333-4178

IOWA

Iowa State Natural Food Associates
Contact: Ron or Val Lucas
RR Box 153
Epworth, IA 52045
(319) 744-3157

KANSAS

Kansas Organic Producers
Contact: Judy Nickelson
P.O. Box 153
Beattie, KS 66406
(913) 353-2414

MAINE

Maine Organic Farmers and Gardeners
Association
Box 2176
283 Water St.
Augusta, ME 04330
(207) 622-3118

MARYLAND

Alternative Farming Systems Information
Center
National Agricultural Library
Room 111
Beltsville, MD 20705
(301) 344-3724

MASSACHUSETTS

Natural Organic Farmers Association of
Massachusetts
21 Great Plain Ave.
Wellesley, MA 02181
(617) 235-1447
(413) 498-2857

New Alchemy Institute
2376 Hatchville Rd.
East Falmouth, MA 02536
(617) 564-6301

Organic Food Production Association of
North America
Contact: Judith Fuller Gillan, Secretary
P.O. Box 31
Belchertown, MA 01007
(413) 323-4531

MICHIGAN

Organic Growers of Michigan
c/o Paw Paw Food Co-op
Contact: Mark Thomas
243 E. Michigan St.
Paw Paw, MI 49079
(616) 657-5934

MINNESOTA

International Alliance for Sustainable Agriculture
1701 University Ave.
Room 202
Minneapolis, MN 55414
(612) 331-1099

Organic Growers and Buyers Association
Contact: Yvonne Buckley
Box 9747
Minneapolis, MN 55440
(612) 636-7933

MISSISSIPPI

Mississippi Organic Growers Association
Contact: Tom Dana
Rt. 1, Box 442
Lumberton, MS 39455
(601) 796-4406

MISSOURI

Ozark Organic Growers Association
Contact: Gordon Watkins
HCR 72, Box 34
Parthenon, AR 72666
(501) 446-5783

NEW HAMPSHIRE

Pest Control for Organic Vegetable
Growers
Cooperative Extension Service
University of New Hampshire
Durham, NH 03824

NEW JERSEY

Natural Organic Farmers of New Jersey
Contact: Al Johnson
RD 1, Box 263
Titus Mill Rd.
Pennington, NJ 08534
(609) 737-9183

NEW MEXICO

Organic Growers Association
Contact: Sarah McDonald, Secretary
1312 Lobo Pl. NE
Albuquerque, NM 87106
(505) 268-5504

NEW YORK

National Organic Farming Association
1152 Merillon St.
Uniondale, NY 11553
(516) 565-2466

Natural Organic Farmers Association
Contact: Pat Kane
P.O. Box 454
Ithaca, NY 14851
(607) 648-5557

New York State NFA
Contact: John J. Nemschick
2274 1st Ave.
Ronkonkoma, NY 11779
(516) 588-2709

NORTH CAROLINA

Carolina Farm Stewardship Association
Contact: Dave Farlow, President
P.O. Box 205
Bynum, NC 27228
(919) 498-7204

OHIO

Organic Crop Improvement Association
(OCIA)
Contact: Betty Kananen, OCIA Administrator
3185 Township Rd., #179
Bellafontaine, OH 43311
(513) 592-4983

Ohio Ecological Food and Farming Association
Contact: Sally Banfield
7300 Bagley Rd.
Mt. Perry, OH 43760
(614) 849-0105

OREGON

Oregon Tilth Certified Organically Grown
Contact: Yvonne Frost
P.O. Box 218
Tualatin, OR 97062
(503) 692-4877

PENNSYLVANIA

Organic Crop Improvement Association
c/o Garden Spot Distributors
Contact: John Clough
438 White Oak Rd.
New Holland, PA 17557
(717) 354-4936

Rodale Institute
222 Main St.
Emmaus, PA 18098
(215) 967-5171

TEXAS

Texas Organic Growers Association
Contact: Ralph Ware, General Manager
Rt. 1, Box 50-B
Thrall, TX 75678
(512) 856-2868

Texas Department of Agriculture
Contact: Keith Jones
P.O. Box 1284
Capital Station
Austin, TX 78711
(512) 463-7602

VERMONT

Natural Organic Growers Association
Contact: Anthony Pollina
15 Barre St.
Montpelier, VT 05602
(802) 223-7222

Vermont Organic Farmers
c/o Golden Russet Farm
Contact: Will Stevens, President
or Enid Wonnacott, Administrator
RD 1, Box 94
Bridport, VT 05734
Will Stevens (802) 897-7031
Enid Wonnacott (802) 434-4435

VIRGINIA

Virginia Association of Biological Farm-
ers
Contact: Diana Bird
Box 252
Flint Hall, VA 22627
(703) 675-3263

WASHINGTON

Washington Department of Agriculture
Contact: Verne Hedlund
406 General Administration Building,
AX-41
Olympia, WA 98504
(206) 753-5042

Tilth Producers Cooperative
1219 E. Sauk Rd.
Concrete, WA 98237
Contact: Ann Schwartz
(206) 853-8449 (home)
(206) 853-8175 (work)

WISCONSIN

Society for Agricultural Training and
Integrated Voluntary Activities Green
Rt 2., Box 242W
Viola, WI 54664
(608) 625-2217

Wisconsin NFA
6616 CTHI
Waunakee, WI 53397
(608) 846-3287

CANADA

Canadian Organic Producers Marketing
Cooperative, Ltd.
Contact: Alfred Moore, President
Box 2000
Girvin, Saskatchewan, SOG 1X0
(306) 567-2810

Canadian Organic Growers
c/o Ecology House
12 Madison Ave.
Toronto, Ontario M5R 2S1
(416) 967-0577

Maritime Sustainable Agriculture Net-
work
Contact: Jane Kehoe or Rod Cann
RR 1
Wolfville, Nova Scotia BOP 1X0
(902) 542-2857

Appendix 2

Consumer Advocate Groups and Environmental Organizations

The following is a list of consumer advocate groups and environmental organizations. Write or call to find out what issues these organizations are specifically involved with, and how these issues are being addressed.

Many of these organizations favor drastic reductions of harmful pesticides and other toxic chemicals in our food supply. Many of these groups are also actively involved in supporting organic methods of farming.

American Vegan Society
501 Old Harding Hwy.
Malaga, NJ 08328
(609) 694-2887

Americans For Safe Food
Center for Science in the Public Interest
1875 Connecticut Ave., NW
Suite 300
Washington, DC 20009
(202) 332-9110

Bio-Integral Resource Center
P.O. Box 7414
Berkeley, CA 94707
(415) 524-2567

Bionomics Health Research Institute
P.O. Box 36107
Tucson, AZ 85740
(602) 297-0798

Citizens For a Better Environment
942 Market St.
Suite 505
San Francisco, CA 94102

EarthSave Foundation
P.O. Box 949
Felton, CA 95018-0949

ECO-NET
3228 Sacramento St.
San Francisco, CA 94115
(415) 923-0900
Provides on-line environmental information

Environmental Defense Fund
257 Park Ave., South
New York, NY 10010
(212) 505-2100

Friends of the Earth
530 7th St., SE
Washington, DC 20009
(202) 543-4312

Greenpeace
1436 U St., NW
P.O. Box 3720
Washington, DC 20007
(202) 462-1177

International Wildlife Coalition
1807 H St., NW
Suite 301
Washington, DC 20006
(202) 347-0822

Mothers and Others for Pesticide Limits
Natural Resources Defense Council
P.O. Box 96048
Washington, DC 20077

National Coalition Against the Misuse of
Pesticides
530 7th St., SE
Washington, DC 20003
(202) 543-5450

National Health Federation
212 W. Foothill Blvd.
P.O. Box 688
Monrovia, CA 91017
(818) 357-2181
FAX (818) 303-0642

National Wildlife Federation
1400 16th St., NW
Washington, DC 20036
(800) 432-6564

Northwest Coalition for Alternatives to
Pesticides
Box 1393
Eugene, OR 97440

Pesticides Action Network
Box 610
San Francisco, CA 94101

Public Citizen
215 Pennsylvania Ave., SE
Washington, DC 20003
(202) 546-4996

Public Voice for Food and Health Policy
1001 Connecticut Ave., NW
Suite 522
Washington, DC 20036
(202) 659-5930

Sierra Club
730 Polk St.
San Francisco, CA 94109
(415) 776-2211

Survival International USA
2121 Decatur Pl., NW
Washington, DC 20008
(202) 265-1077

Vegetarian Resource Group
P.O. Box 1463
Baltimore, MD 21203
(301) 366-VEGE

World Resources Institute
1709 New York Ave., NW
Washington, DC 20006
(202) 638-6300

Worldwatch Institute
1776 Massachusetts Ave., NW
Washington, DC 20036
(202) 452-1999
FAX (202) 296-7365

World Wildlife Fund
Dept. ZB40
1250 24th St., NW
Washington, DC 20037

Appendix 3

Detoxification Resources

The American Natural Hygiene Society, founded in 1948, by Dr. Herbert M. Shelton, is a non-profit organization whose purpose is to educate people on how to lead a toxic-free lifestyle. The American Hygiene Society, based in Tampa, Florida, houses the Herbert Shelton Library. The library contains thousands of volumes on Natural Hygiene. Some volumes date back to the 1830's.

The American Natural Hygiene Society is the largest Natural Hygiene organization in the world, with members in more than twenty countries. The society has local chapters in the United States and Canada, holds seminars and annual public conventions, and publishes the monthly journal *Health Science*.

For membership fees and the locations of Natural Hygiene chapters nearest you contact:

> The American Natural Hygiene Society
> P.O. Box 30630
> Tampa, FL 33630
> (813) 855-6607

The Canadian Natural Hygiene Society is a non-profit organization whose motto is, "To further good physical and mental health by the promotion of all aspects of natural living." The Canadian Natural Hygiene Society sells a large selection of Natural Hygiene books and audiotapes. The Society has chapters in Toronto, Montreal, Peterborough, and Kitchener. For membership fees and the locations of chapters nearest you contact:

> The Canadian Natural Hygiene Society
> P.O. Box 235, Station T
> Toronto, Ontario M6B 4A1
> CANADA
> (416) 781-0359

Dr. Keki R. Sidwa is President of the British Natural Hygiene Society. Dr. Sidwa singlehandedly introduced Natural Hygiene to Britain more than forty years ago. He deserves much credit for the tremendous work he has done in advancing principles of healthy living.

The British Natural Hygiene Society publishes a quarterly journal which is sent to members. For further information and membership fees contact:

> Dr. Keki R. Sidwa
> British Natural Hygiene Society
> Shalimar Retreat - 3 Harold Grove
> Frinton-On-Sea, Essex C0139BD
> ENGLAND
> 011-44-25-567-2823

Dr. Alec Burton, President of the Australian Natural Hygiene Society is very active in the Natural Hygiene movement. He and his wife, Nejla, are popular speakers at health seminars and conventions worldwide. The Burtons are directors of Arcadia Health Centre, an internationally acclaimed Natural Hygiene retreat near Sydney. For further information contact:

Dr. Alec Burton
Dr. Nejla Burton
Australian Natural Hygiene Society
31 Cobah Rd.
Arcadia, New South Wales 2159
AUSTRALIA
011-61-2-653-1115
011-61-2-653-2678

Founded by Jo Willard, Natural Hygiene Incorporated is a non-profit organization devoted to advancing Natural Hygiene. Natural Hygiene Inc. maintains a research department that provides information on subjects related to toxic-free living, and publishes the official magazine of the organization, *Journal of Natural Hygiene.*

Jo Willard has discussed Natural Hygiene over the airwaves for more than 18 years. Her radio show is heard on WPKN in Bridgeport, Connecticut. For further information and membership fees contact:

Jo Willard
Natural Hygiene Inc.
P.O. Box 2132
Huntington Station
Shelton, CT 06484
(203) 929-1557

Natural Hygiene Practitioners

The following Certified and Associate Professionals are primary care doctors licensed and/or legally practicing in their state, country, or territory, who are members in good standing of the International Association of Professional Natural Hygienists (IAPNH) and as such agree to accept and abide by the Association's Principles of Ethics and Standards of Practice.

Those listed as Certified members include the founders of the Association and those subsequent members who have successfully completed an internship (or its equivalent) in Natural Hygienic care with an emphasis on Fasting Supervision and are certified by the IAPNH as Specialists in the Application of Fasting Supervision and Natural Hygienic Care. The American Natural Hygiene Society assumes no responsibilities for fees charged, health care rendered, or guidance provided.

Certified Members

Charisse Basquin, D.C.
2900 St. Paul Dr., #219
Santa Rosa, CA 95405

Gerald Benesh, D.C.
2050 Rockhoff Rd.
Escondido, CA 92026
(619) 747-4193

John Brosious, D.C.
18209 Gulf Blvd.
Redington Shores, FL 33708
(813) 392-8326

Alec Burton, D.O., D.C.
Nejla Burton, D.O.
Arcadia Health Centre
31 Cobah Rd.
Arcadia, New South Wales 2159
AUSTRALIA
011-61-2-653-1115
653-2678

Ralph C. Cinque, D.C.
Hygiea Health Retreat
439 East Main St.
Yorktown, TX 78164
(512) 564-3670

Theodora Coumentakis, M.D.
Palaion Polemiston 30
Gylfada, Attici
GREECE
962-2387

Ronald G. Cridland, M.D.
Health Promotion Clinic
9955 Younge St., Suite 102
Richmond Hill, Ontario L4C 9M6
CANADA
                    (416) 737-0810

William Esser, D.C.
Esser's Health Ranch
P.O. Box 6229
Lake Worth, FL 33466
                    (407) 965-4360

Douglas F. Evans, D.O.
P.O. Box 78
Culburra Beach, New South Wales
2540
AUSTRALIA
                    044-472-081

Alan Fraley, D.C.
Alan Goldhamer, D.C.
Alec Isabeau, D.C.
Jennifer Marano, D.C.
Center for Chiropractic
 & Conservative Therapy
4310 Lichau Rd.
Penngrove, CA 94951
                    (707) 792-2325

Alan Immerman, D.C.
Immerman Chiropractic Center
5743 East Thomas Rd., Suite 2
Scottsdale, AZ 85251
                    (602) 946-1597

Philip Martin, D.C.
15 Ridge Hill Dr.
Toronto, Ontario M6C 2J2
CANADA
                    (416) 482-2340

Frank Sabatino, D.C., Ph.D.
Regency Health Resort and Spa
2000 S. Ocean Dr.
Hallandale, FL 33009
                    (305) 454-2220

D. J. Scott, D.C.
P.O. Box 361095
Strongsville, OH 44136
                    (216) 671-5023

Keki R. Sidwa, D.O.
Shalimar Retreat - 3 Harold Grove
Frinton-On-Sea, Essex C0139BD
ENGLAND
                011-44-25-567-2823

Andrew Vitko, D.C.
17023 Lorain Ave.
Cleveland, OH 44111
                    (216) 671-5023

Associate Members

Norman Allard, D.C.
323 North Wisconsin St.
Gunnison, CO 81230
                    (303) 641-4044

Stanley S. Bass, D.C.
3119 Coney Island Ave.
Brooklyn, NY 11235
                    (718) 648-1500

Antonio Brito, M.D.
Aptdo. 5098
48080 Bilbao
SPAIN

Paul W. Carlin II, D.C.
711 Bay Area Blvd., Suite 130
Webster, TX 77598
                    (713) 332-1111

Pierre Cloutier, D.C.
Chiropractic-Optometric Clinic
132 Saint-Jean Baptiste
Chateauguay, Quebec J6K 3B2
CANADA
                    (514) 691-1102

Jacques Dezavelle, D.C.
1118 Second St.
Encinitas, CA 92024
(619) 436-5151

Greg Fitzgerald, D.O., D.C.
1/31-33 Geralle St.
Cronulla, Sydney 2230
AUSTRALIA
523-2108

Stephen Forrest, D.C.
430 Monterey Ave., Suite #2
Los Gatos, CA 95030
(408) 358-2188

Dale John Frazer, D.O.
36 Kiwong St.
Yowie Bay, New South Wales 2228
AUSTRALIA

Joel Fuhrman, M.D.
412 Benedict Ave.
Tarrytown, NY 10591
(914) 332-4090

Douglas N. Graham, D.C.
Club Hygiene
105 Bruce Ct.
Marathon, FL 33050
(305) 743-3168

Thomas K. Hand, D.C.
3676 Richmond Ave.
Staten Island, NY 10312
(718) 984-5869

Guy Harris, D.O.
4-12-4 Minami
Nagasaki, Toshima-ku
Tokyo, 171
JAPAN

Steve Nelson, D.C.
7340 Ulmerton Rd.
Largo, FL 33541
(813) 535-7754

Anthony J. Penepent, M.D.
P.O. Box 886
Long Beach, NY 11561
(516) 486-6469
(212) 239-9582

David L. Reichel, D.C.
330 West Main St.
Perham, MN 56573
(218) 346-2330

Philip C. Royal, D.C.
2607 De La Vina St.
Santa Barbara, CA 93105
(805) 569-1702

Leslie H. Salov, M.D.
The Vision & Health Center
Rt. 4, Box 186
Whitewater, WI 53190
(414) 473-7361

Detoxification Spas

Those looking to detoxify in a supervised program, may want to check out Natural Hygiene Health Spas. These spas serve mostly fruits and vegetables. Meals are high in fiber, low in fat, low in sugar, and low in sodium. Foods served are designed to rid the body of toxins. All of the spas listed offer personalized fasting programs. In addition to fasting, some of these spas offer juice diets and other methods of detoxification.

Although all Natural Hygiene Health Spas offer detoxification programs, the atmosphere, services provided, and costs vary from spa to spa. Write or call for brochures. The spas listed are coed.

Arcadia Health Centre
31 Cobah Rd.
Arcadia, New South Wales 2159
AUSTRALIA
          011-61-2-653-1115
                    653-2678

Club Hygiene
105 Bruce Ct.
Marathon, FL 33050
          (305) 743-3168

Esser's Health Ranch
P.O. Box 6229
Lake Worth, FL 33466
          (407) 965-4360

Health Oasis
HC 33, Box 10
Tilly, AR 72679
          (501) 496-2364

Hippocrates Health Institute
1443 Palmdale Ct.
West Palm Beach, FL 33411
          (407) 471-8876

Hygiea Health Retreat
439 Main St.
Yorktown, TX 78164
          (512) 546-3670

Hygiea-West
2607 De La Vina St.
Santa Barbara, CA 93105
          (805) 569-1702

Regency Health Resort and Spa
2000 S. Ocean Dr.
Hallandale, FL 33009
          (305) 454-2220

Scott's Natural Health Institute
Box 361095
Strongsville, OH 44126
          (216) 671-5023
          (216) 238-6930

Shangri-La Health Resort
P.O. Box 238
Bonita Springs, FL 33923
          (813) 992-3811

The Umpqua House
7338 Oak Hill Rd.
Roseburg, OR 97470
          (503) 459-4700

BIBLIOGRAPHY

Barone, Don., et al. *The Doctors Book of Home Remedies*. Emmaus, Pennsylvania: Rodale Press, 1990.

Bieler, Henry G. *Food Is Your Best Medicine*. New York: Random House, 1965.

Bower, John. *The Healthy House*. New York: Carol Communications, 1989.

Carson, Rachel. *Silent Spring*. Cambridge, Massachusetts: Houghton Mifflin Company, 1962.

Consumer Guide. *Complete Book of Vitamins and Minerals*. Lincolnwood, Illinois: Publications International, Ltd., 1989.

Cooper, Robert K. *Health and Fitness Excellence*. Boston: Houghton Mifflin Company, 1989.

Curtis, Helena. *Biology, Fourth Edition*. New York: Worth Publishers, 1984.

Dadd, Debra Lynn. *The Nontoxic Home*. Los Angeles: Tarcher, 1986.

Nontoxic and Natural. Los Angeles: Tarcher, 1984.

Davies, Stephen and Alan Stewart. *Nutritional Medicine*. New York: Avon Books, 1990.

Diamond, Harvey and Marilyn. *Fit for Life*. New York: Warner, 1985.

Living Health. New York: Warner, 1987.

Giehl, Dudley. *Vegetarianism: A Way of Life*. New York: Harper and Row, 1979.

Golos, Natalie and Frances Golos Golbitz. *Coping With Your Allergies*. New York: Simon and Schuster, 1986.

Gross, Joy. *The 30-Day Way to a Born-Again Body*. New York: Rawson, Wade Publishers, Inc., 1980.

Hazzard, Linda Burfield. *Scientific Fasting: The Ancient and Modern Key to Health*. New York: Grant Publications, 1927.

Hoffman, Ronald L. *7 Weeks to a Settled Stomach*. New York: Pocket Books, 1991.

Isselbacher, Kurt J., et al. *Harrison's Principles of Internal Medicine, Ninth Edition*. New York: McGraw-Hill, 1980

Kime, Zane R. *Sunlight*. Penryn, California: World Health Publications, 1981.

Kimmel, Dean D. *The Dieter's Directory: A Comprehensive Guide to Diets*. New York: Corbin House, 1990.

Kowalski, Robert E. *The 8-Week Cholesterol Cure.* Revised edition. New York: Harper and Row, 1989.

Macfadden, Bernarr. *Fasting for Health.* New York: Macfadden Book Company, 1934.

Marlin, John Tepper and Domenick Bertelli. *The Catalogue of Healthy Food.* New York: Bantam, 1990.

McDougall, John A. *McDougall's Medicine.* Piscataway, New Jersey: New Century, 1985.

The McDougall Plan. Piscataway, New Jersey: New Century, 1983.

Mindell, Earl. *Unsafe At Any Meal.* New York: Warner, 1987.

Vitamin Bible. New York: Warner, 1985.

Newbold, H.L. *Mega-Nutrients For Your Nerves.* New York: Berkley Books, 1981.

Null, Gary. *Clearer, Cleaner, Safer, Greener.* New York: Random House, 1990.

Oswald, Jean A. *Yours For Health: The Life and Times of Herbert M. Shelton.* Franklin, Wisconsin: Franklin Books, 1989.

Randolph, Theron G. *Human Ecology and Susceptibility to the Chemical Environment.* Springfield, Illinois: Charles C. Thomas, 1962.

Rinzler, Carol Ann. *Are You At Risk.* New York: Facts On File, 1991.

Shelton, Herbert M. *Fasting Can Save Your Life.* Chicago: Natural Hygiene Press, 1964.

Health For The Millions. Chicago: Natural Hygiene Press, 1968.

Human Life: Its Philosophy and Laws. Oklahoma City: How To Live Publishing Company, 1928.

The Hygienic Care of Children. Chicago: Natural Hygiene Press, 1970.

The Hygienic System, Vol.II. San Antonio: Dr. Shelton's Health School, 1956.

The Hygienic System, Vol.III. San Antonio: Dr. Shelton's Health School, 1963.

An Introduction to Natural Hygiene. Pasadena, California: Health Research, 1954.

Natural Hygiene: Man's Pristine Way of Life. San Antonio: Dr. Shelton's Health School, 1968.

Superior Nutrition. San Antonio: Dr. Shelton's Health School, 1971.

Smith, Lendon. *Feed Your Kids Right.* New York: Delta, 1979.

Tracy, Lisa. *The Gradual Vegetarian.* New York: Evans, 1985.

Trop, Jack D. *Please Don't Smoke in Our House.* Chicago: Natural Hygiene Press, 1976.

Warmbrand, Max. *Add Years to Your Heart.* New York: Whittier Books, 1956.

Whitaker, Julian M. and June Roth. *Reversing Health Risks.* New York: G.P. Putnam's Sons, 1988.

Wolinsky, Harvey and Gary Ferguson. *The Heart Attack Recovery Handbook.* New York: Warner, 1988.

Wright, Jonathan V. *Dr. Wright's Guide to Healing With Nutrition.* Emmaus, Pennsylvania: Rodale Press, 1984.

Zamm, Alfred V. and Robert Gannon. *Why Your House May Endanger Your Health.* New York: Simon and Schuster, 1980.

ABOUT THE AUTHOR Dean D. Kimmel, a medical research writer, holds a Bachelor of Science degree from the University of the State of New York at Albany. He is a health consultant, lecturer, and the author of two highly acclaimed health and fitness books, *The Untold Truth About Fatness* and *The Dieter's Directory.* An avid hiker and photography enthusiast, the author resides in New York City.

Index

A

acetylcholine, 26
additives, iv, 35, 37
adolescents, 21
adrenaline, 26
aerosol sprays, 19
agribusiness interests, 7
agricultural chemicals, 7, 9
Agriculture Department, 10
air, xi, xiii, 8, 15, 17, 19-20, 30
air fresheners, 19-20
Alar, 1-2 , 4
alcohol, 19, 24, 28
alcoholic beverages, 24, 28-30
aldicarb, 2-4
Alka-Seltzer, 17
Allard, 130
allergic reactions, 28-30
aluminum, 36, 91-92
Alzheimer's disease, 36, 92
American Natural Hygiene Society,
    127, 129
Americans for Safe Food, 1
analgesics, 24
anemia, 91
anger, 26, 32-33
animal consumption, 6
animal fat, 27, 32
animal products, 24-25, 90, 92
animals, 6, 24, 63, 90
antacid, 17
anti-oxidant vitamins, 85, 90
anti-oxidants, 85-86
antibiotics, 5-6, 9
apple growers, 2
apple industry, 2
apple juice, 2, 75, 99, 110-111, 114
apple sauce, 2, 99, 110
apples, 1-2, 35-36, 38-41, 43, 45, 47,
    57, 63-66, 68-69, 89, 95, 97, 99,
    100-101, 103, 106, 110, 113-114
Arcadia Health Centre, 128
arteries, 17-18, 25-26

arterioles, 24
arteriosclerosis, 18
arthritis, 29
artificial coloring, 5
artificial flavors, 91-92
artificial sweeteners, 27
asbestos, 27
ascorbic acid, 86-87
aspartame, 27
asthma, 16, 30
asthmatics, 15
atherosclerosis, 25
Auerbach, 4
Australian Natural Hygiene Society,
    128

B

B vitamins, 86, 90
B-complex vitamins, 30, 86
back pain, 20
bacon, 27
baking soda, 20
bananas, 2-3, 38-39, 43, 45-47, 59,
    65, 79, 87, 89, 101
Basquin, 129
Bass, ix, 130
bathing, 15, 16
beans, 25, 27, 31, 36, 42-44, 47, 51,
    56, 58, 60-61, 67, 75, 86-89,
    95-98, 103, 105-107, 109-112
beef, 6-7, 27, 85, 100, 103-104,
    108-109, 111, 114-115
beef liver, 85
beef producers, 7
beer, 28
Benesh, 129
benzopyrene, 27
beta carotene, 25, 27, 32, 86, 90
biotin, 87
birth defects, 6-8, 10, 24

C